Life of a Warrior

KEEPING THE PROMISE

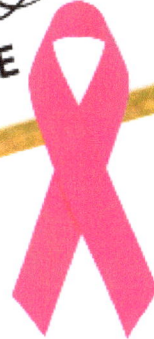

Demetris Price

Life of a Warrior
"Keeping the Promise"
By: Demetris Price

ISBN: 979-8-9855858-0-3 (Paperback)
ISBN: 979-8-4210162-0-5 (Paperback)
ISBN: 979-8-9855858-6-5 (Hardcover)
ASIN: B09S1F4SB6 (eBook)

Library of Congress Control Number: 2022901898

Photography: Raymond Jackson
Cover Design and Layout design by Quisqueyana Press

To order additional copies of this book, visit QuisqueyanaPress.com/Demetris-Price or Amazon.com or contact:

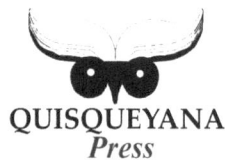

QUISQUEYANA
Press

Quisqueyana Press
Poway, California, USA
info@quisqueyanapress.com
www.quisqueyanapress.com

"If ye have faith of a grain of mustard seed, you can move mountains"

– Quinton Jason "Chef Q."
from Matthew 17:20

CONTENT

Pag.

09 Dedication

11 Introduction

12 June Warriors
13 "Who are June Warriors?"
14 Where it all Starter June McCarty

16 Warriors
17 Demetris Price – President
18 David Garcia – Vice-President
19 Donald P. Price Jr. – Sergeant of Arms
20 Lisa Thompson – Secretary
21 Sean Joseph – Treasurer & DJ
22 Raymond Jackson - Treasurer & Publications
23 Kenneth Thompson – Chaplain
24 Joseph Griffin – Event Administrator
25 Deborah Green – Décor Administrator
26 Reka Wilkerson – Public Relations
27 Santana Howard – Event Cook
28 Vernon Bell
29 Dontroy Thorne
30 Joycelyn Duplessis
31 Keith Augustine

CONTENT

Pag.

32   Marlon Jackson (Mowop)

33   Vanessa Richard

34   Ramonia Jackson Jenkins

35   Talmadge Scott

36   Ivory Haley Jr.

37   Devin M. Price

38   Eric Augustine Jr.

39   In Remembrance but Never Forgotten

40   June Marie Wallace Price McCarty.

       Sept. 01, 1950 - April 3, 2011

42   Quinton Irvin Jason.

       April 6, 1965 – Sept. 26, 2020

44   Zenobia Williams Garcia

       May 21, 1961 - Dec. 29, 2009

46   Tanya Rose.

       August 31, 1968 – Sept. 25, 2017

48   Many Others

51   Poem: The True Warrior

54   The Rule Basketball Team

55   Past, Present and Future Committee

80   Acknowledgment

81   Afterword

83   Call to Action

I would like to dedicate this book

to our brother, Quinton Jason,

and all the Warriors we lost.

He fought a good fight, and he never gave up.

"Have a little faith", his words.

INTRODUCTION

This book is about ordinary people, hard workers. Some started as supporters to end up as survivors, living and loving life, keeping the promise, given to their loved ones. Some battling cancer, some lost their battle, others supporting the cause, and those who are telling their stories for encouragement to never give up. It tells the stories of the loved ones on the sideline, their hurts and their struggles. Cancer is hard, but you don't have to fight it alone. The stories shared help those struggling to know there's hope, information about awareness, and resources.

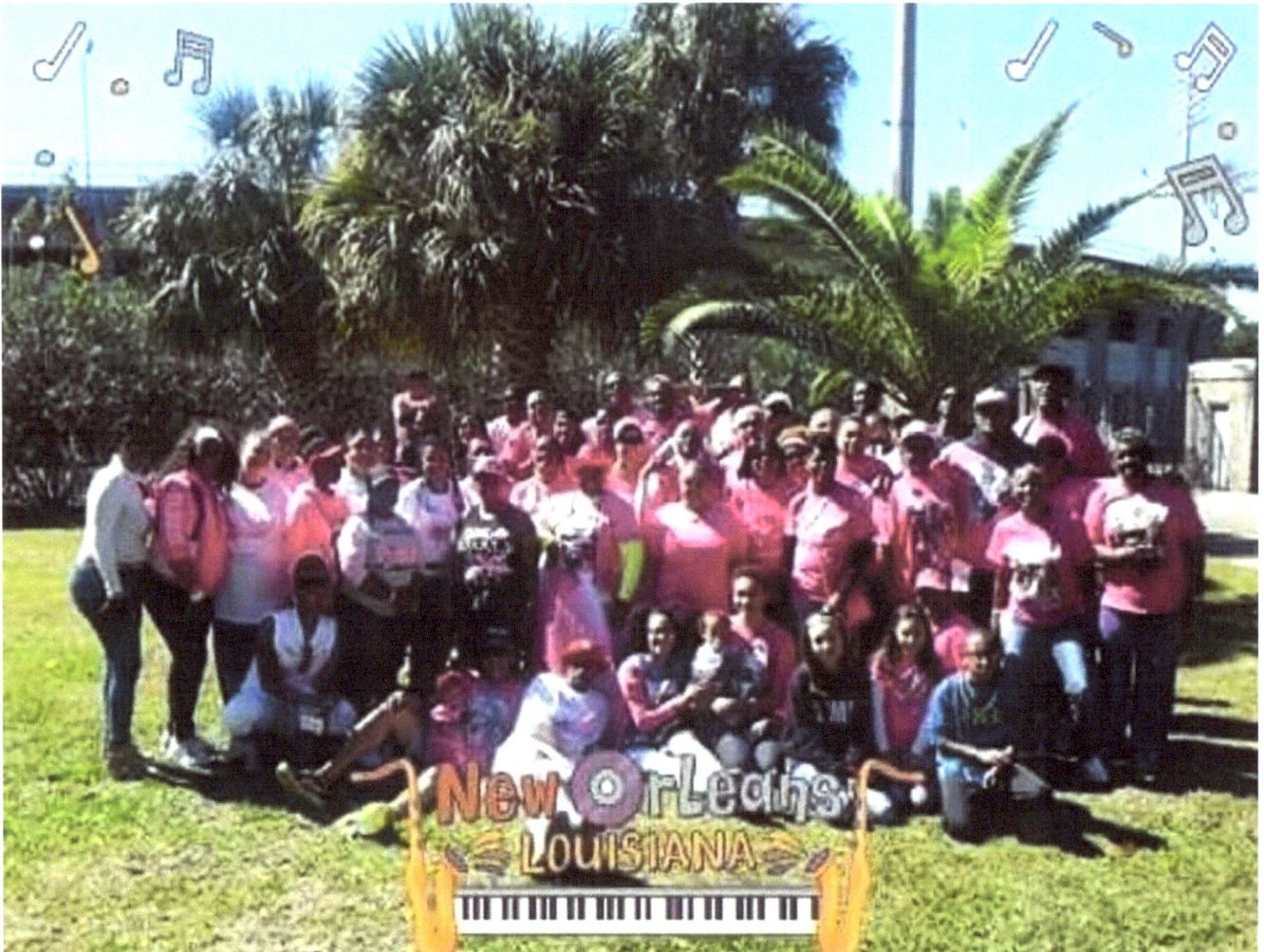

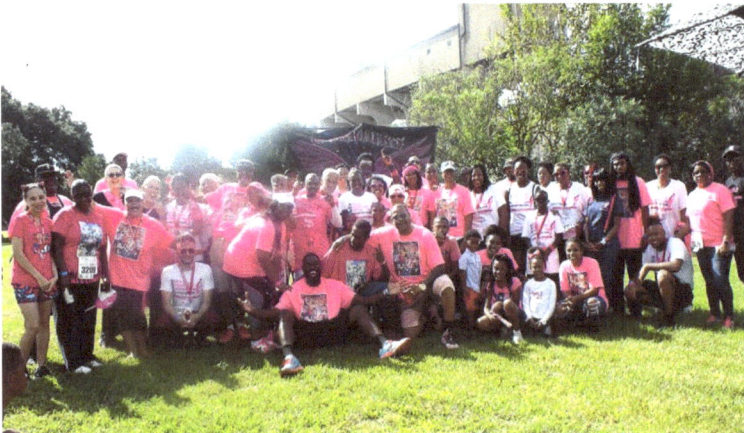

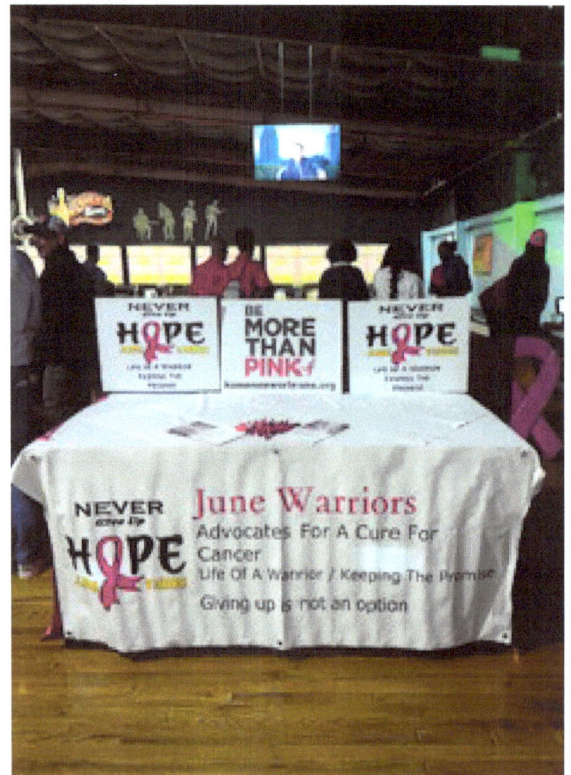

June Warriors a group of people bonded together through love, hope and friendship, making a difference, and helping in supporting and finding a cure for Cancer.

ADVOCATES FOR A CURE FOR CANCER

WHO ARE JUNE WARRIORS?

We have an amazing team of twelve committee members and a race team of about 247 members who are devoted advocates for a cure for cancer, Warriors for life. We are that support group, family member, friend. We don't let you fight cancer alone. We pledge to do whatever it takes to advocate and educate the community on awareness of all cancer. We are the voice of those who can't fight. We are brothers, sisters, husbands and wives, daughters, sons, children of loved ones battling this awful disease.

Friends in our group were being diagnosed. We had men come out to cook and do whatever it took to support the cause. One day, one of the men found out he had cancer, then another, then another. We started focusing on men can get cancer too and started campaigning and advocating the cause "Men Can Get Breast Cancer". It wasn't until 2019 when it really got the recognition it deserved, and advertisement came out with some of the big names in the city of New Orleans, The Westbank, Algiers, and people out of town came far and dear to support the cause, and we are so thankful for this. We have pictures of someone from some part of New Orleans, whether its uptown, downtown are central city, showing love for what we do.

90% of all the proceeds made are always taken in by June Warriors to the organizations for cancer research and Susan G. Komen to organization for research to find a cure for cancer, the other remaining 10% of proceeds go into helping us be able to give the events around the city. What is not known is that the committee members hustle and give out of their own pockets along with donations from friends to put on some of the elaborate events around the city. June Warriors have had some of New Orleans' local finest artist and musicians perform at their events, Angela, "Oh I Believe Bell", Lil Soulja Slim, A 'Darryl Bell, Ben E. Hunter Folk singer, Rochelle Cook R&B Songstress, Queen Keilla and The Kings, Fi Yi Yi Mandingo Warrior, Spy Boy, Al Polite, who lost his wife to cancer and joined our group. The Zulu Walking Warriors with one of June's best friends supporting the cause, Jimmy and The Zulu Tramps, Spy Boy Nell with the Wild Magnolia and Fi Yi Yi with The Baby Dolls and many more.

At times, we put out more than we take in, but this group is committed to the cause. We have learned along the way, and we are doing better with how we prepare for future events. We are Warriors; we stand strong behind what we do and have never had a failed event. We do not fail, and we never give up. June Warriors have two big events a year, one honoring a male and female survivor and two volunteers of the year. The other one on race day. June Warriors gives events throughout the year to raise money, which is turned over in October, and we begin again from the first week of December. I am proud of the people in this organization, and all their accomplishments, honors, and awards. We started out as friends, but if you pull any Warrior on the side, I bet they say, "We are family".

WHERE IT ALL STARTED

JUNE McCARTY

JUNE WARRIORS'S FOUNDER

Meet June and Moss McCarty. June was a two-time cancer survivor. She fought a good fight and lived the promise to never give up. As a true warrior, she started the team we all know today as June Warriors. In 2011, she lost the battle to cancer but passed the torch down to her supporters to keep the promise and to never give up and inspire others to tell their stories.

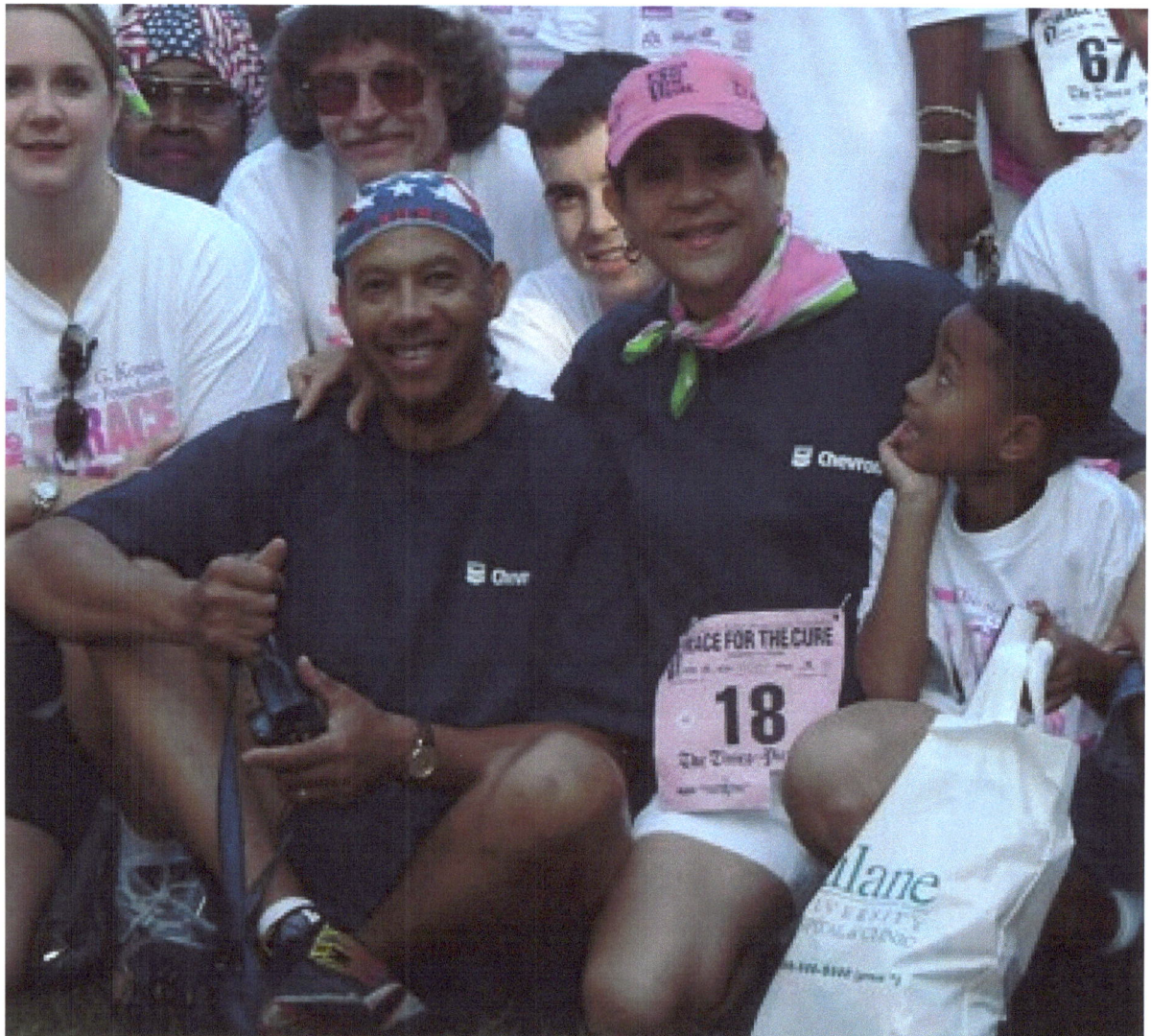

We are not survivors, we are Warriors.

BEEN THERE

SURVIVOR

BEAT THAT

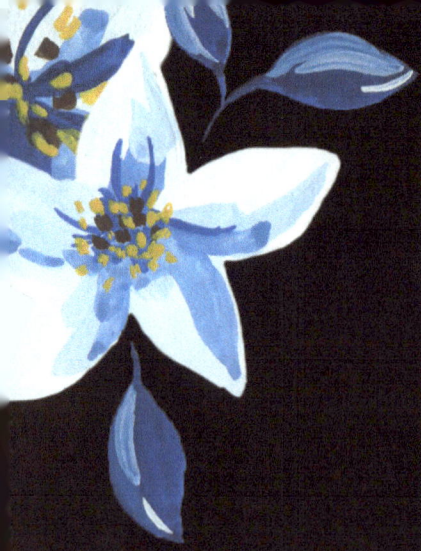
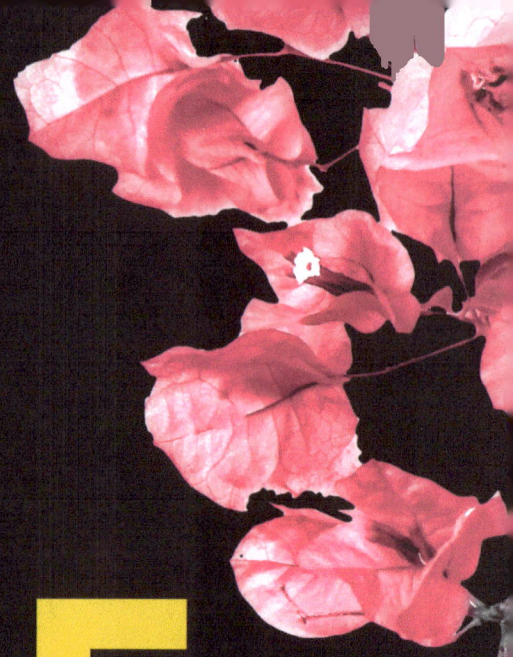

JUNE
Warriors

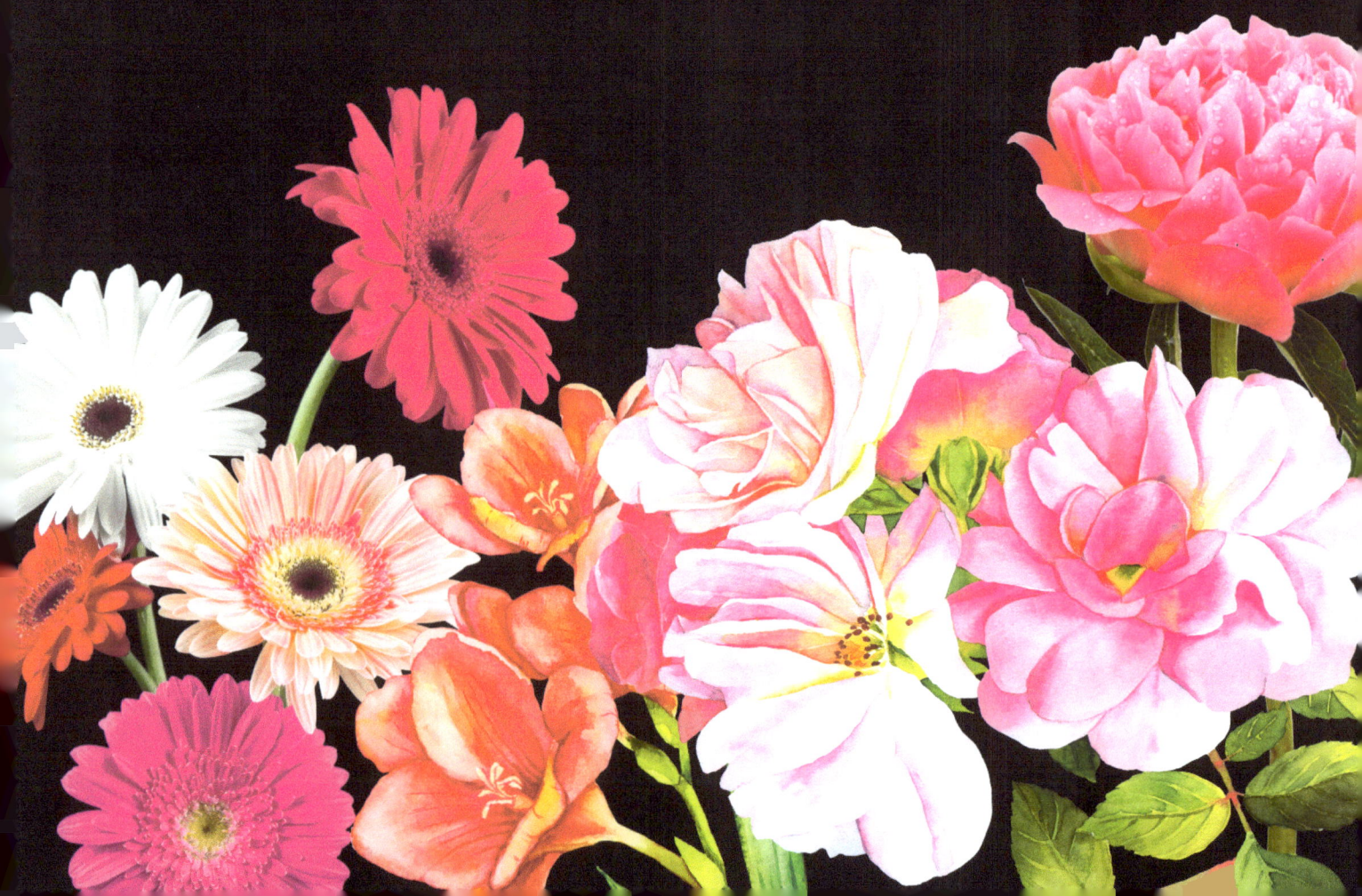

Demetris Price

President

Advocate for a cure for cancer, I PLEDGE to help find a cure, and giving up is not an option. I started this organization with my husband Donald Price and David Garcia after his mother June Marie McCarty died after battling cancer. David lost his wife Zenobia Garcia to breast cancer. We used to go to City Park to race for a cure and support all loved ones fighting this battle while celebrating the memory of those who lost the fight. June was a big part of the organization along with her husband Moss McCarty. My whole family along friends would come out and support the cause. Our family combined was hit hard with cancer as I lost my grandmother, Francis Melson to breast cancer, and my grandfather, Prince Bernard Melson to prostate cancer and myself with cervical cancer.

I did not know how much work was involved until the torch was passed down to me. We have met a lot of people along the way. It taught me a good support team is key to survival, along with faith and hope. Our motto is "We never give up".

Through prayer, faith, love, and the testimony of our survivors have given so many hopes. Cancer is not a death sentence, and we are here to share and give hope and to let those going through it know they are not alone. My story is different, I don't consider myself and never called myself a survivor, my word was always Warrior. Friends would ask, I would say, I'm a Warrior. Only three knew, not even my family. I say a survivor survives, day by day, but a warrior fight to the bitter end. That's my motto, that's why we call ourselves Warriors. We won't stop fighting until we find or those who we pass the torch too find a cure for cancer. Ask any of our members, they will say I was once a survivor, now I am a Warrior.

I have a testimony, God has sent his guardian angels to look over me, Doctor said no more kids, my life or the baby. I would have chosen the baby. I love kids, but my husband said no. I wasn't leaving him to take care of three boys and be by himself. Four bad car accidents and fought off three attackers. Yes, I'm a Warrior. I was taught by a strong woman, Selina Ford Horton to be strong, to put your trust in God. I had Donald who was my strong arm. My faith that with God "All things are possible."

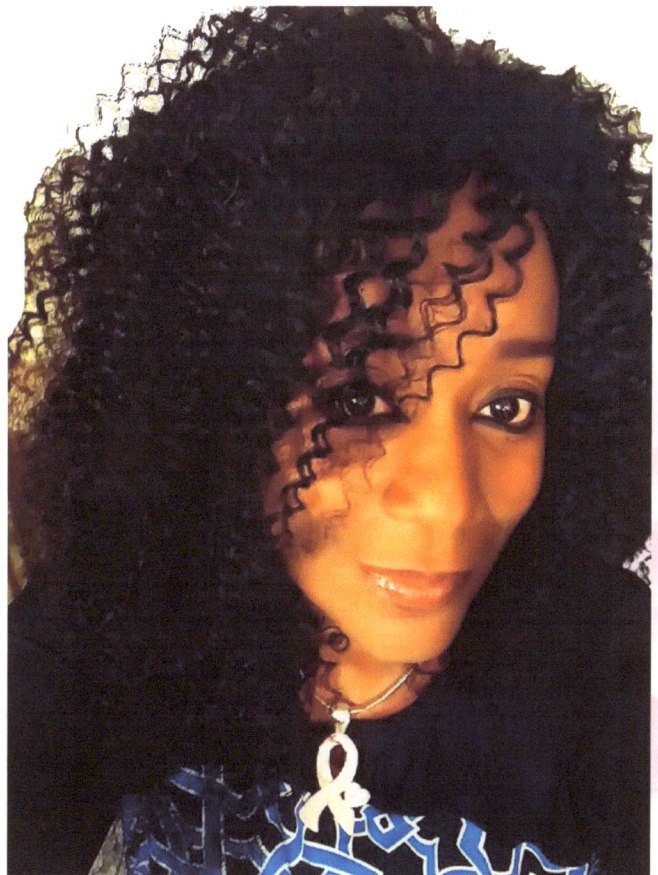

David Garcia

Vice President

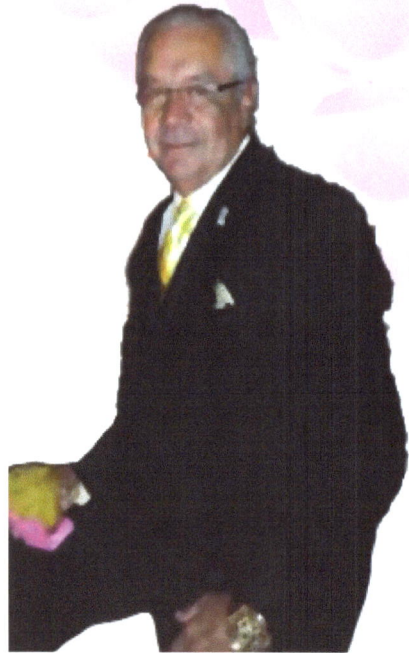

My name is David Garcia, vice president of June Warriors. I am an advocate for breast cancer. I lost my beautiful wife, Zenobia A.W. Garcia, to breast cancer. She was a true Warrior, and she fought it for two years. Zenobia passed away in December 2009. We have 4 children, Danielle, Jackie, David, and Marianne. It was hard at first; I did not know which way to turn. My daughter, Jackie helped a lot. She took care of her little sister, Marianne, who was 10 at the time. She helped through high school and college. If not for her, I don't know what I would have done. Jackie is still by my side today. What a blessing! And she gave me a bundle of joy, my grandson.

I was not prepared for life without my better half. Some days, I didn't know where to turn. My best friend, Terry Williams, got me to church every Sunday. My walk with God got stronger. This is what I needed, and I eventually joined Pentecostal Baptist Church under the leadership of Pastor Lionel Davis. It is a wonderful congregation and pastorship. You need a strong support team because there are so many unanswered questions. This is not taught; these are life lessons. You must have faith, you must be a believer, you must never lose hope. If it had not been for the Lord, guiding my footsteps and strengthening me, where would I be?

The fellows, The Rule basketball team, family, and friends helped me along the way. I started the Susan G. Komen Race for A Cure with my friend Donald and his wife when his mother passed. We became a trio alone with the guys, boiling, frying, parties, events; you name it. We did it on prayer and donations. Through the years, we have seen so many of our brothers go home to be with the Lord.

We advocate for men because men don't go to get checked, men try to not tell their story. We are supposed to be strong; we got this. We cannot tell our loved ones we are sick; we cannot show a sign of vulnerability. For some men, this is not so, until it's too late. We don't go to the doctors; we don't stay informed on health issues. We are too afraid to find out the truth. I have learned that being silent is not the way early detections save lives. This I can testify to because we had two members in our group who did this. We are family. June Warriors. We have a strong, loving, and caring committee.

We are here for one another, and we are warriors to the end. We have come out of our pockets many times for the cause without any hesitation. I want to thank a wonderful lady, our president, Demetris Price, for all the hard work she does and the committee. We are committed to finding a cure. This is my promise to my beautiful wife, Zenobia, living a life of a Warrior, all for the cause.

Donald P. Price Jr.

Sergeant of Arms

June McCarty was my mother. Donald Phillip Price was my father. Being the only child, it was hard to lose both parents to this awful disease. Cancer has no name on it. I have lost a lot of friends and family members. I never thought I would lose my mother in the prime of her life. She was gone too soon. Cancer takes everything away from you. Life is not the same and you never stop grieving. So, imagine after fighting that battle, you turn around to do it all over again with your dad. I am married with three sons and a grandson, but that is a hole that cannot be filled. You need a strong support group and I have that with June Warriors and family, but through it all, my walk with God got closer. My faith got stronger, for if it were not for God, I could not have made it. It tests your strength, and I can testify I was not always strong. I did not give up, and I think my parents would be proud of the man I am today.

I started this group with my wife Demetris, and my best friend David after my mom passed away. We supported her in the Race for A Cure with Susan G. Komen, and when she passed, we kept going. A few of the fellows and The Rule Basketball Team often get together to throw fundraisers in support of a cure. All men and one woman, my wife. We decided to get her some help, and that's how June Warriors was founded. We now have four women and a host of friends and family who volunteers. In our group of men, we realized we were not being checked, going to the doctors, being in the know about health issues, so we combined them both and started advocating for both. Men get cancer too. Who knew years later we would have so many men in our group being diagnosed with this disease, once an advocate to a survivor? Never lose your faith in what God can do. We do not know His will, His plan for our life, but that is a journey I am ready to take. My spiritual walk with God.

Thankful for His Grace.

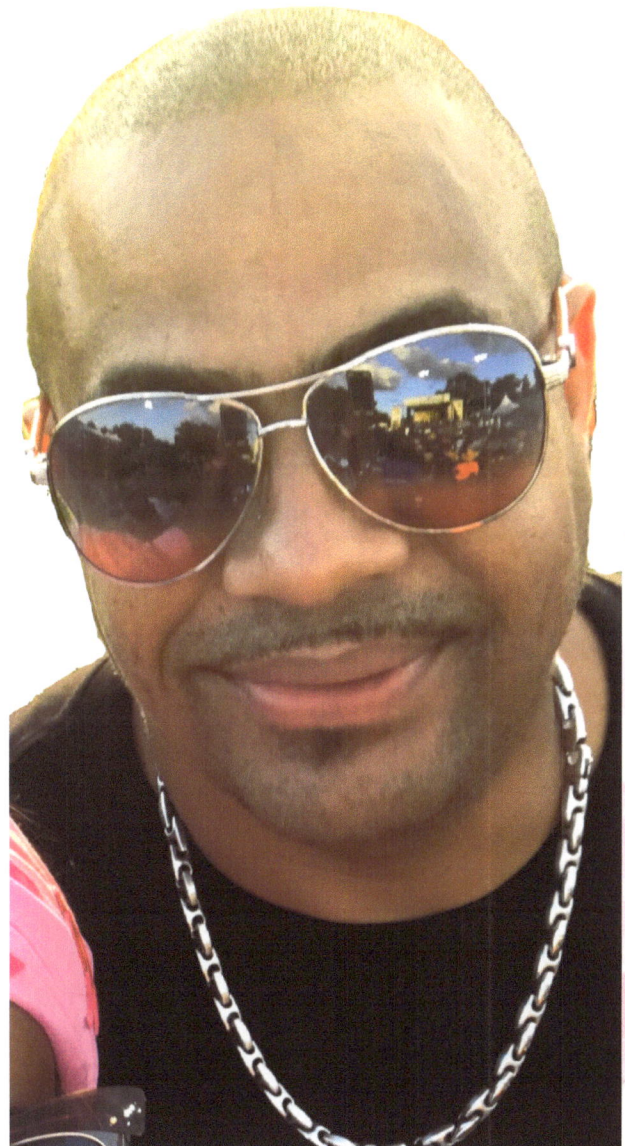

Lisa Thompson

Secretary

meet every challenge and come out on top. I know God has favor on our committee. I feel immensely proud to be a part of June Warriors knowing that I am helping to fight breast cancer, encouraging those that are on the battlefield, celebrating those that have won the battle, and comforting the family of those that have lost the battle. I am continuously praying for the cure.

I joined June Warriors about four years ago. For many years, my husband was involved with them in fundraising activities and the cancer walk. Unfortunately, I was unable to attend many events, except the one year when he asked if I would help to set up for a fundraising activity before I go to work. I helped to set up but did not go to work because I was moved to see how much effort was involved in this group to battle this disease and plus; I had so much fun helping with the kid's booth. Later that year, I made sure I attended the breast cancer walk. When I approached one of the race booths, the attendant asked if I would like to write down and wear any names of cancer survivors, those that lost the battle, or were in the middle of the battle. As I began to write down the names of family and friends, I realized just how much this disease has affected so many in my life.

The following year, at one of June Warriors' events, Demetris asked if anyone was interested in being on a committee for June Warriors. I signed up and attended several meetings and was later asked to become the secretary. Since then, I have been the secretary for June Warriors and have helped plan and participated in many breast cancer awareness fundraising activities. Every year, the challenges become greater and greater, but for some reason, June Warriors always

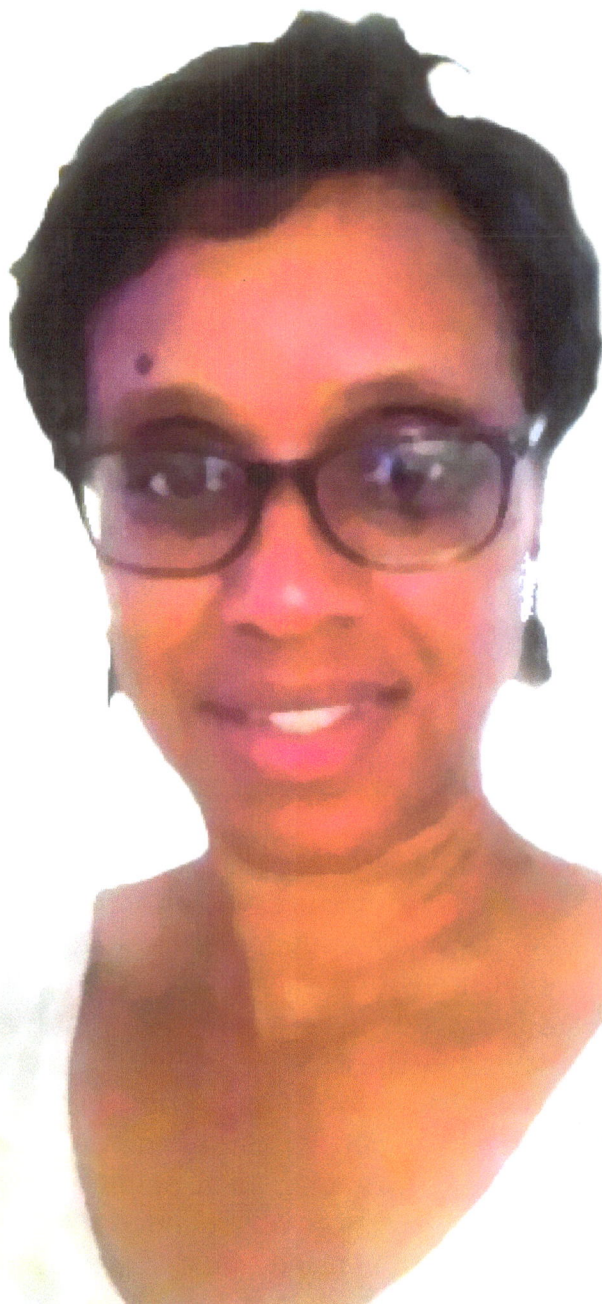

Jean Joseph

Treasurer & DJ

As a youngster, I never paid much attention to the ills of cancer. My family was relatively healthy, so I didn't think about it much. However, as I grew older, it became more prevalent as I watched my father-in-law succumb to prostate and intestinal cancer. Since then, various friends and family members have either lost the good fight or have been diagnosed with various cancers, including breast cancer. As a man of faith, husband, and father of four (Including three daughters), I have become a Warrior in the fight against breast cancer and breast cancer awareness.

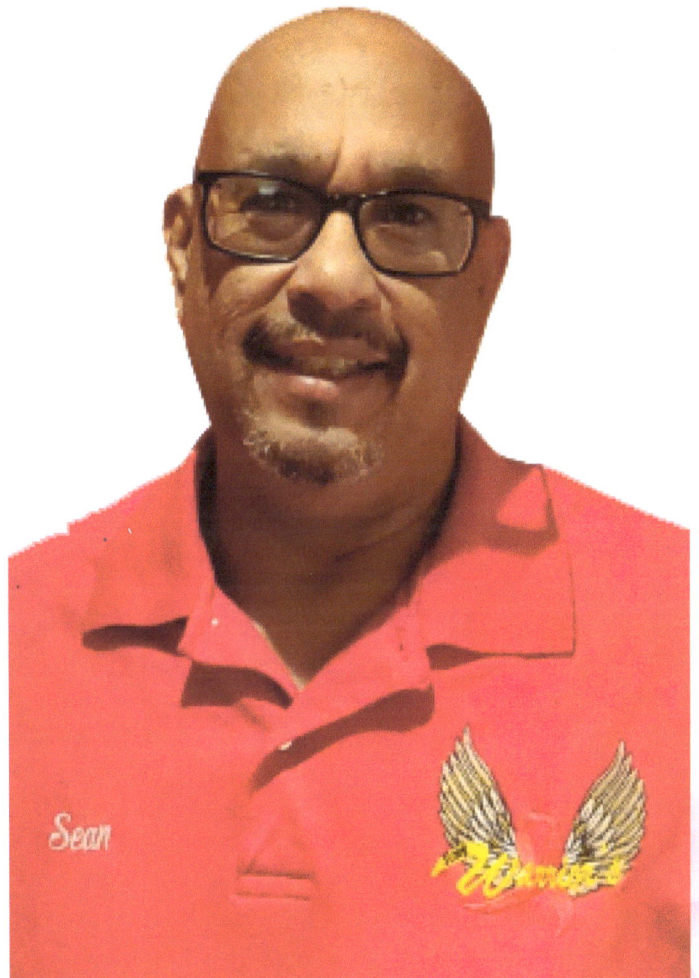

Raymond Jackson

Treasurer & Publications

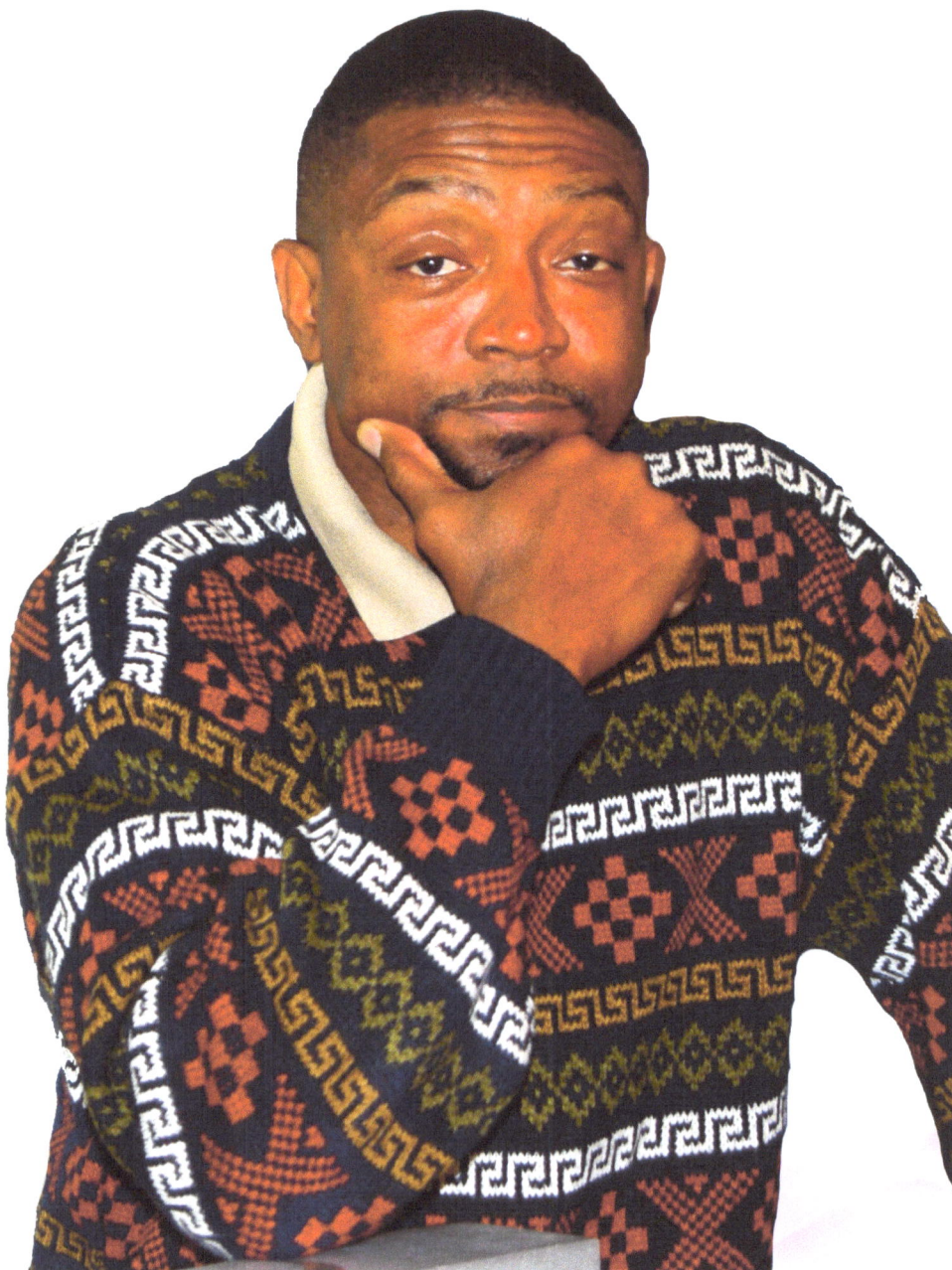

From the time I was a child, I have known someone in my family that had their life turned upside down with the devastation of a diagnosis of cancer. As a child, all I could do was worry and pray. The loss of a family member from a child's point of view is as distressing as the diagnoses. Despairing hopelessness and fear are just some of the apprehensions.

The loss of my grandfather to lung cancer made me want to do more than pray for those stricken with this awful disease. Breast cancer is one of the most devastating diagnoses a woman can undergo. I have four sisters and know firsthand just how it can overwhelm someone's life. As an adult, I was given the opportunity to do more than worry about who in my family or friends was next. The June Warriors gave me just the avenue to make a difference. Working with a group of like-minded, goal oriented, and focused people permit me to give more than my concerns, worries, and prayers.

Kenneth Thompson

Chaplain

My name is Kenneth Thompson, but everyone calls me Meekey. I was affiliated with Da Rule basketball team when I found out they were taking part in the annual breast cancer walk. We walked in honor of my team member, Donald Prices' mom, Mrs. June, who was battling breast cancer. I participated in the breast cancer walks until I was unable to walk the long distance. At that point, I began to grill oyster on the day of the event along with my son. A few years later, a fundraising committee was formed in honor of Mrs. June, called June Warriors. My wife and I volunteered to become members of the committee, but I was later appointed as the Grill Master and Chaplain.

Over the years, I have committed my time to raising money to help find a cure. My experience in the food industry and tireless efforts at many fundraising events have made June Warriors successful in helping to find the cure for breast cancer. My knowledge about cancer and the impact it has on your life was little to none prior to joining June Warriors. Now I see that a cancer diagnosis goes beyond the person with the disease. It affects family and friends. Recently, two of my brothers were diagnosed with cancer. Now, I know the battle is not only theirs but also, my battle too. My battle is to do whatever it takes to give them hope and encouragement to keep them uplifted in spirit, to stay on the battlefield, and fight with all their hearts to win no matter how many times they get knocked down mentally and physically.

I have learned this by hearing the experience of breast cancer survivors at our annual Pink and White end of year event. June Warriors have given me the avenue to become an advocate for the cure and to encourage and give hope to those who are going through this horrible disease.

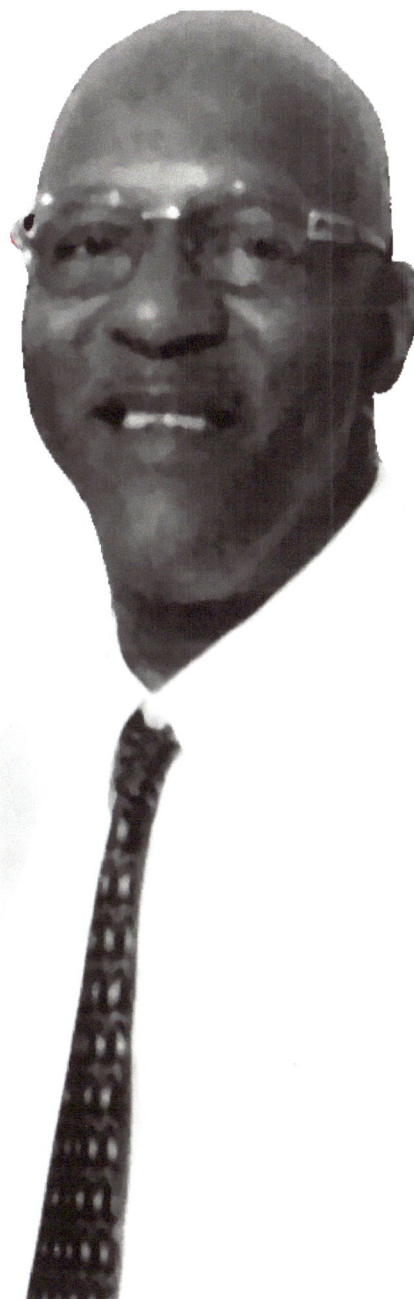

Joseph Griffin

Event Administrator

I have been with the Warriors family from the beginning. I was a volunteer and made my way up to the committee. I have no problem with advocating for the cause and have done everything and anything to building the set, to taking down the set. It brings a warm comfort to my heart when everything is in place and you know, with the help of God, I was a big part of this.

In 2017, I was the volunteer of the year. What an honor. We all started out as just friends together, losing some along the way, but as they say, "true friendship never dies." We are a family. I am a warrior for life, committed to helping find and supporting the cause.

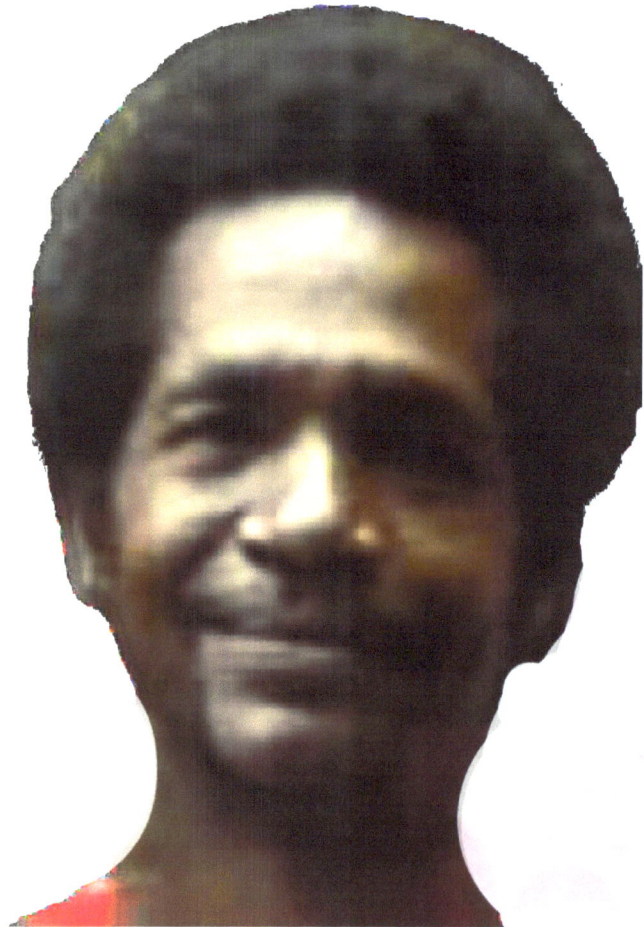

Deborah Green

Decor Administrator

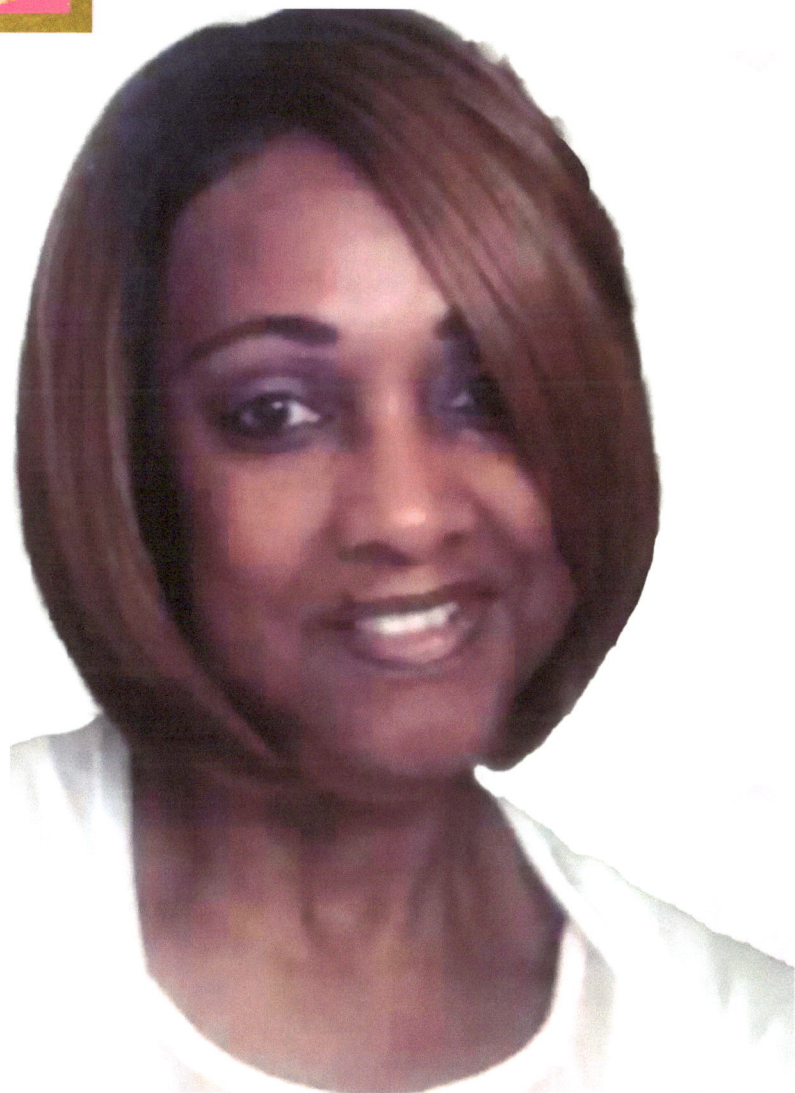

One of the reasons I decided to become a June Warriors member is because of the way they always do something to help cancer survivors. I started out by going to their functions with my sister, Lisa, and brother -in-law, Kenneth Thompson. I loved the activities, and I said to myself, "wow, this is awesome". They are doing something that I have a passion for, and that is helping those that are in need. Also, I love the fact that they all love and care for each other. They are family. So, I decided that this is a team that I would love to be a part of, June Warriors. Supporting those that are in need.

Love you guys!

Reka Wilkerson

Public Relations

Hi, my name is Reka Wilkerson. I began my journey with June Warriors in 2017 after attending one of their committee meetings and fell in love with the passion and dedication that the Warriors had for not just breast cancer, but for all types of cancer. I set through this meeting and instantly knew what I had to do. Back in 1997, I was stationed in Hawaii when I got the news, my dad had 6 months to live due to stage 4 pancreatic cancer. I was absolutely devastated! That's when I found out the seriousness of this disease. I immediately flew to the United States to take care of my dad!

Six months of pure hell and six months to the date; he was gone! Just like that, I had seen firsthand how cancer invades and attacks the human body. It was literally gruesome. Since then, I've lost more family and friends to some sort of cancer. Therefore, I joined the June Warriors team in their fight against cancer. And I must mention…. I found another family with this close-knit team. This sums up why I am and choose to be a Warrior!

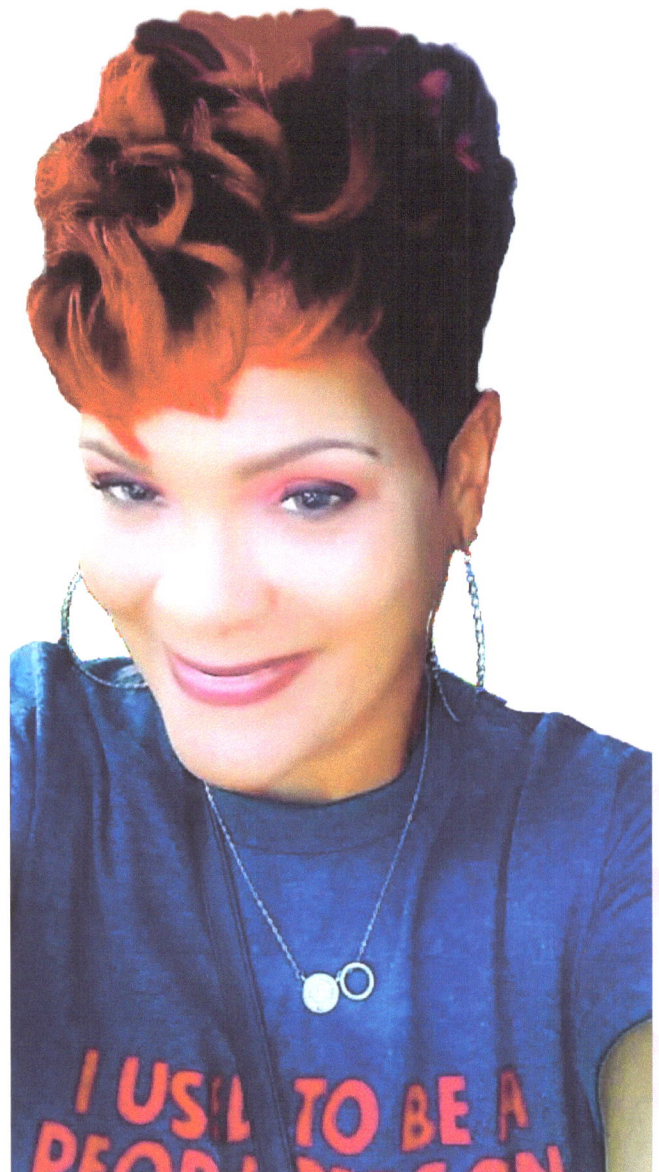

Santana Howard

Event Cook

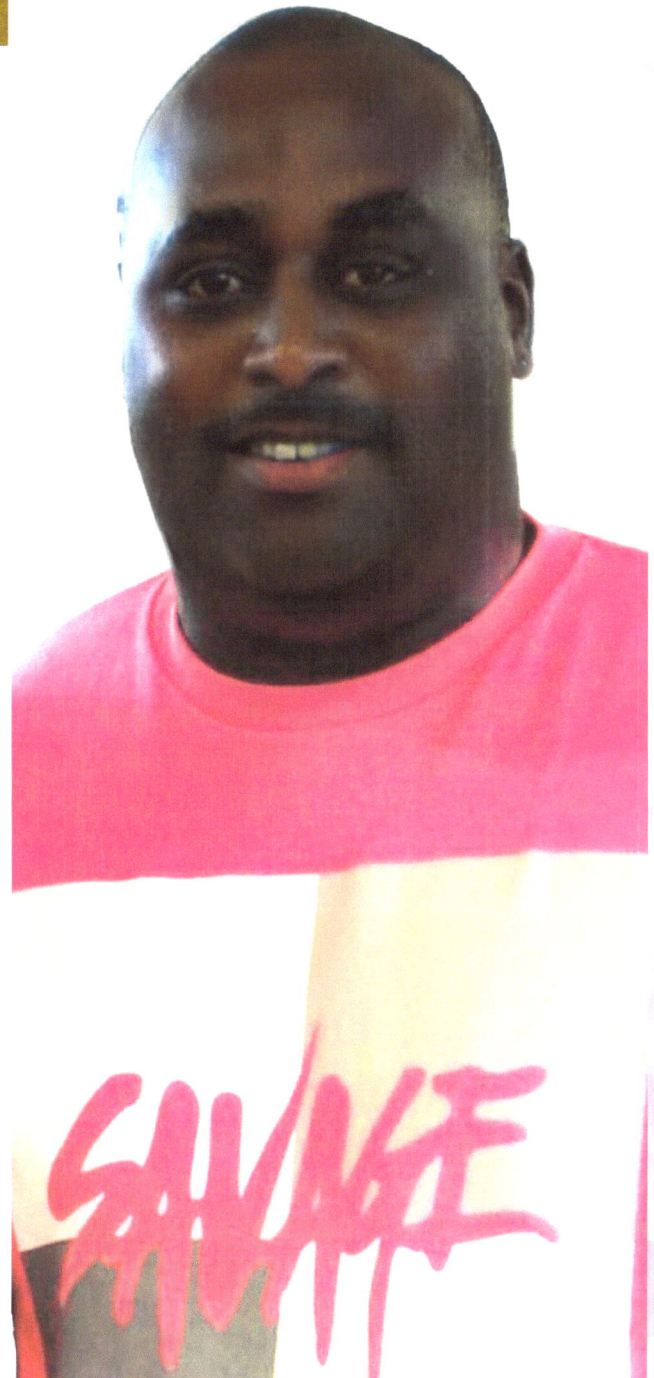

Hi, my name is Santana, and I became associated with June Warriors through my good friend, David Garcia. I have met some great people through this organization. I love the way they give back to the community by educating everyone about the importance of yearly mammogram checkups to help prevent breast cancer. With such a great cause like that, I will help in any way I can. You will usually find me boiling seafood, with all the sides.

I'm a Warrior.

Vernon Bell

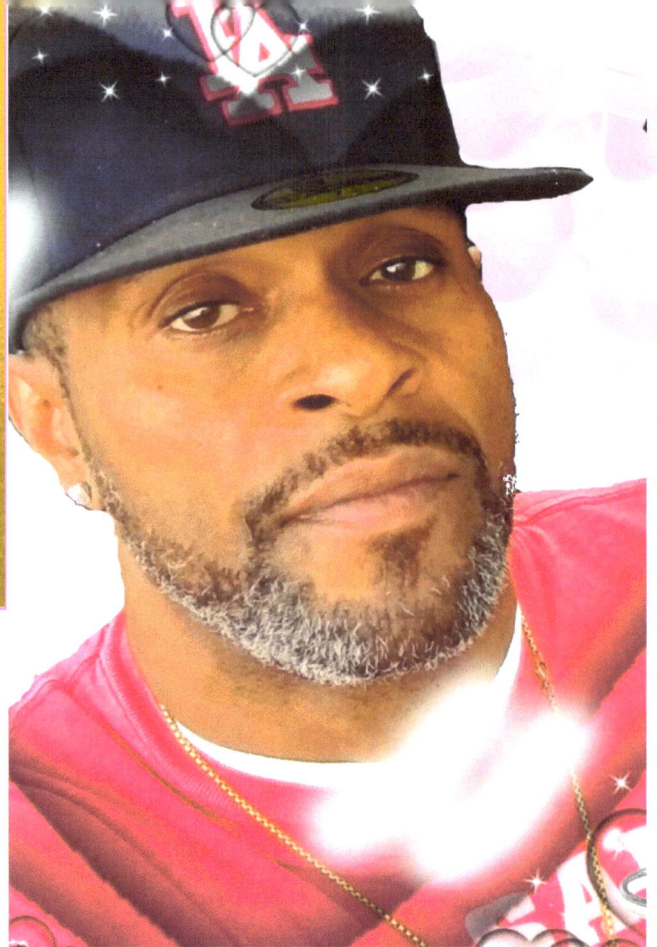

My life changed after I was diagnosed. I remember waking up one morning with pain in my arm. After checking, I noticed I had a lump under my arm. I ignored it and as time went on; I noticed it began to grow. Sometimes I had pain, sometimes just discomfort. I didn't want to alarm anyone, I'm not sure why, but as time went on, it became larger. I tried to hide it, but the pain and discomfort became unbearable. I showed it to a friend of mine, Demetris, one day at work. She was so mad that I hid it without telling anyone or going to the hospital; she asked me to go to the doctor to get checked. I did, but truth be told, it was a fatty tissue. I believed what they said and began to live my life as they said it would go away. It didn't. I tried to hide it. Days passed by and it got bigger. I couldn't put down my arm. I asked Demetris to help me put on my sweater, as it was starting to be noticeable. When she saw how big it was, she stated again that I should go get checked. I did.

What a shock to be told you have cancer and need to start treatment. The initial shock hadn't taken place until I had to start chemo. I went to the hospital and was told I wasn't going home; they needed to start immediately. My first treatment went well. The second one was pretty much the same as the first. I was like, okay, I can do this, but one day I went, and treatment didn't go well. My brother, John, called my friend and asked her if she had seen me. Good thing I told them where I was going, because I had a reaction and was placed on lockdown. This cause me to be uncomfortable with taking any more treatments, but I continued to take them and live my life one day at a time.

Finding out you have cancer is life changing. You wonder if this is the end. How am I going to get through this? My sisters and brothers were there for me. You must have a support group, because depression sets in if you try to handle it all alone, but never lose faith, because many nights when I sat alone, my mind wondered, but the God I serve never left my side and His mercy and grace is why I can say I am here. One day at a time, it is life changing, but it makes you grateful for what you have and the surrounding people. I'm a Warrior and giving up is not an option.

Dontroy Thorne

Da Rule basketball team member to Survivor Now Warrior.

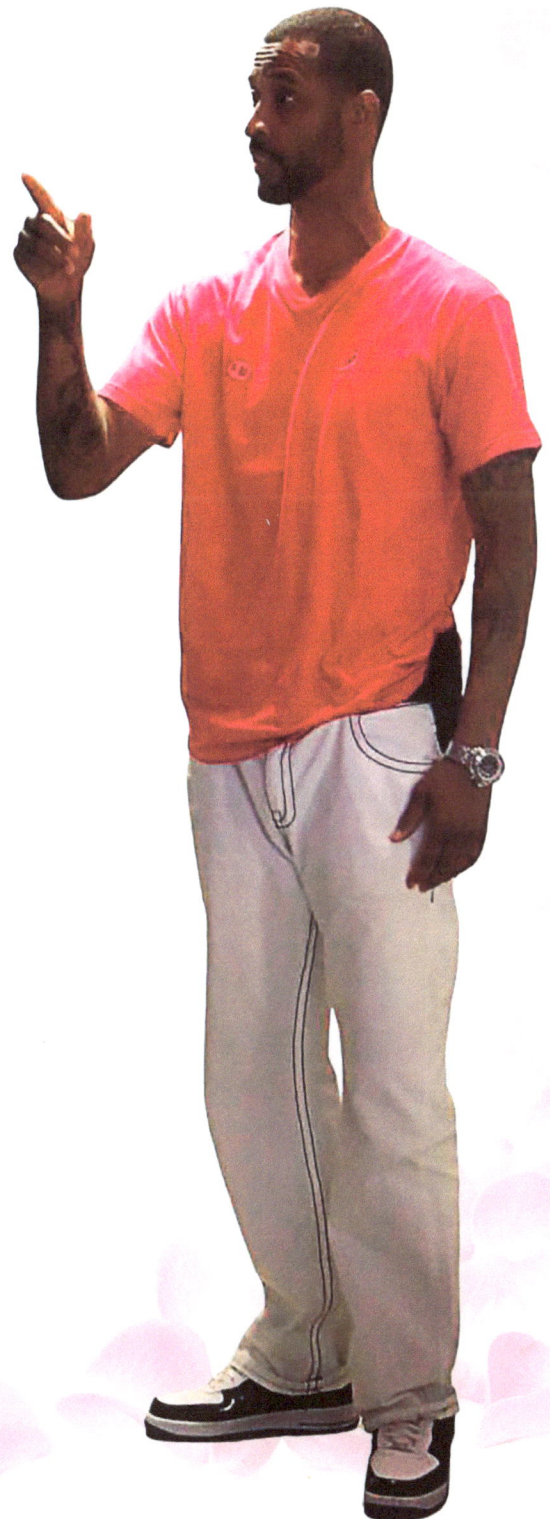

Joycelyn Duplessis

First, I would like to thank my Lord and savior, Jesus Christ, for giving me a platform today to stand on and tell you all that He is the one who has given me life and more abundantly. Without God, I do not know where I would be.

Second, I'm grateful to each one of my family members, friends, and support group June Warriors, who have been traveling alongside me since I have been on this journey. I was born in 1962. I was raised in New Orleans, Louisiana by my amazing mother and father and 10 siblings. I am blessed with 3 sons and 8 grandchildren. I am a graduate of a high school in the New Orleans public school system, an infant/toddler childcare provider, earning a CDA through Penn State University. I love traveling, meeting new people, and just embracing "Life".

I was diagnosed with stage 3 breast cancer in 2015 and went through it with the help of the Lord. Since then, other than teaching, I have started two small businesses of my own. I am an independent Paparazzi Jewelry Consultant and make door wreaths. I love making things with my hands! I am so thankful that God has given me a second chance. I am forever grateful that I have found my purpose, blessings flowing!

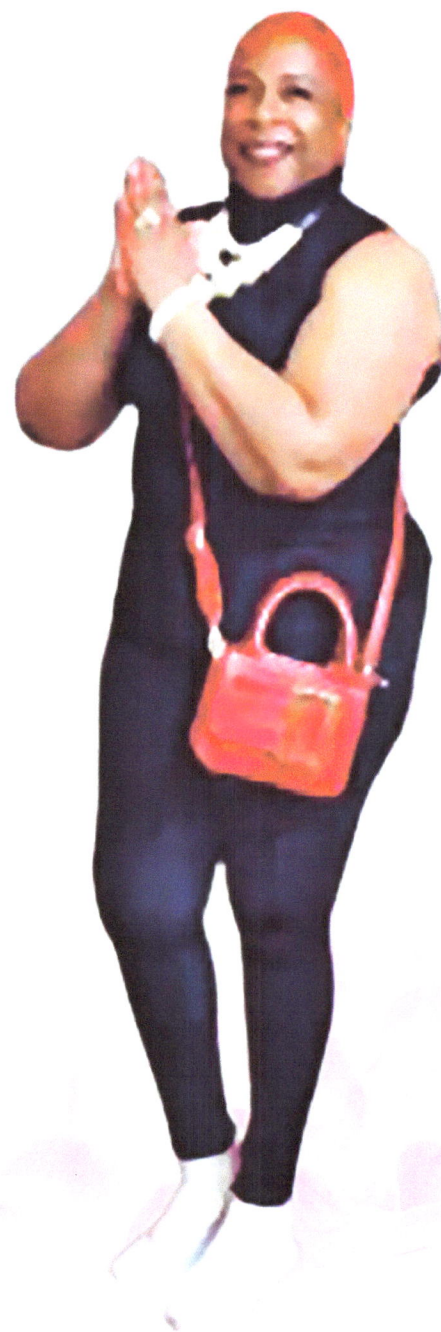

Keith Augustin

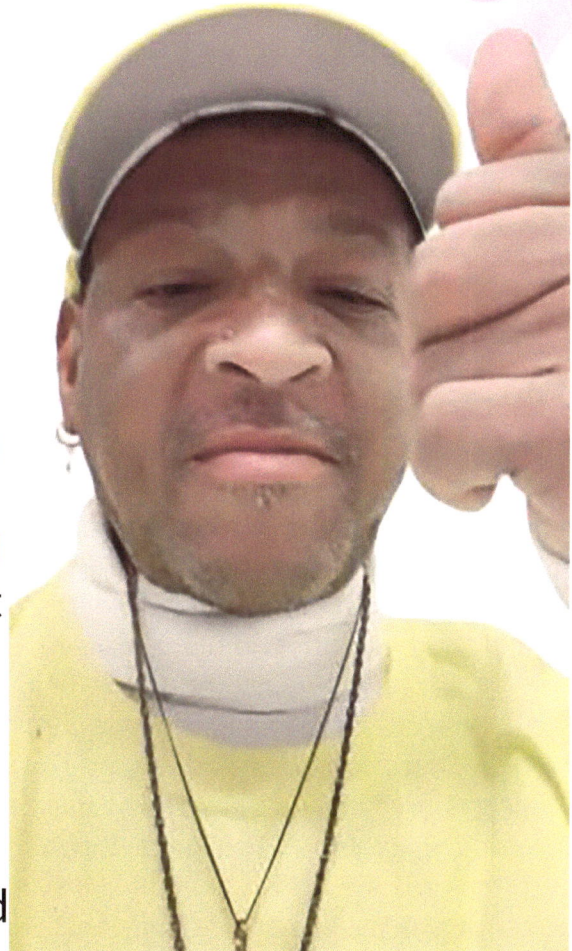

I kept going to the doctor because I was worse, and they kept telling me nothing was wrong with me and said I had chronic bronchitis. I went to work as normal in the morning and some minutes into work; I started coughing up blood. So, I ran from my job on Bourbon street to University Hospital. The doctor came to see me in the room and told me I had stage 4 cancer with less than 24hrs to live.

My brother passed away a day before my surgery. I'm now cancer free after 3yrs, I whipped that cancer in the ass. I fought every day. Now at me. I have my own home again, after I lost everything, my job of 40yrs, but believe me, God is good. I am a very great witness to His work. I am a miracle, and I am God's child.

Marlon Jackson

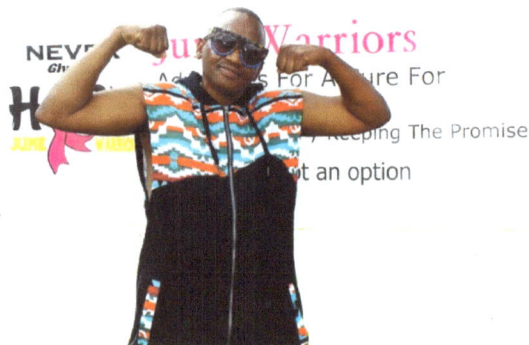

My name is Marlon Michael Jackson (Mowop). In September 2013, I had an abscess under my left arm. I thought it was a burl. I told myself I needed to go to the hospital to get checked, but I didn't go. One day, I notice my hand had become swollen. I was like, "this is not okay", I need to go now. I waited a few days trying to diagnose myself and wind up with two blood clots in my arm. I went to Ochsner Hospital to get help. I wanted them to admit me and get to the core of the problem, but the doctor had to go through proper procedures and was amazed at the size of the knot. I asked her not to lance it, but she ordered the procedure to be done anyway, experimenting on me like a guinea pig. That was how I felt. They kept me in the hospital, then discharged me and gave me medication to take home. While recovering, I received a call telling me that a daughter to a friend of mine has died from an aneurysm. This made me panic.

So, I decided to go for a second opinion at the University Hospital. This was nothing but God, I'm telling you. The doctors asked if they performed a biopsy on me. I replied "no"; but one was done immediately. They came back in the room and told me, "Mr. Jackson, you're diagnosed with diffuse large B cell lymphoma, a form of cancer." I replied, "No way, I don't have cancer. I am a basketball player and a good one for my age. I am a legend, an icon in Algiers." This was what my crazy self-told the doctor. I also told him that I had a game in three days. My oncologist said, "Mr. Jackson, I am going to have problems with you, Mr. Jackson. Most patients I give this news to would ask how long they had to live; not I have a game in three days." That dumbfounded me, and I started my treatment immediately.

Early detection saves lives. I know I am a fighter; both of my parents were diagnosed with cancer. My mother was given two years but lived nine. My father, on the other hand, was diagnosed with lung cancer right after me. During his treatments, he wouldn't stop smoking cigarettes and so it defeated the purpose.

When I received a call from my brother telling me my father lost the battle, I was hurt, but it made me more determined not to give up. When I was diagnosed, I told myself, "Mowop, you're going to beat this cancer and you're going to play basketball again at a higher level." I had hope, faith and I believed it. I told Doctor Castillo that he was going to tell other cancer patients how positive I was through the process. I was going to make my parents proud of me.

When I was going to my sixth treatment, my oncologists, Doctor Castillo and Ruiz, both came into my room and said, "Mowop, this is your last treatment. We are not detecting anymore cancer anywhere." I cried on the spot, and both hugged me. That's a moment I will never forget. God is an awesome God. This I know, this I believe. I thank God every single day after I beat that old cancer. Demetris and Donald introduced me to June Warriors Breast Cancer Team, and I have been connected ever since. I am cancer free from the year 2012. Now, I am playing ball in two leagues, so you tell me, what can God not do. I am humble and thankful. He's a miracle worker, healer and provider.

Vanessa Richard

God wants me to testify to His goodness. My mother was a breast cancer warrior. I was supposed to get mammograms every 6 months. Year after year, my mammogram came back negative, so I stopped getting the exams. It was nobody but God that led my mind to get my annual mammogram. Why not? It was free.

April 2017, my mammogram showed something. After 4 different mammograms, including a 3-D mammogram, it was discovered that I had breast cancer. I didn't have to have a mastectomy (removal of the breast); however, on July 5th, I had a lumpectomy surgery (Removal of the lump). Another surgery on August 16, of resizing, due to pre-cancer cells developing.

The key it was caught early, early, early. Initially, chemotherapy nor radiation was required, but due to genetic reasons (my mom, aunt, and 3 cousins,) 4 chemo, and 6 weeks of radiation was ordered. I started my 1st chemotherapy on October 30th, and by the second one my hair came out, looking like beetle juice (Y'all know how I felt about my hair, but I thank God for life). I completed chemotherapy on January 2, 2018.

I started radiation on February 12, finished on March 19th. After I got the results of the radiation on Tuesday April 24th, I was discharged by the radiologist. Thank God! Again. My cardiologist gave me a praise report and said she'll see me in November 2018.

I will say thank God over and over again for His goodness. I volunteer to direct a choir at a local church on 4th Sunday, or when they need me. I feed the hungry (when money permits) and try to do for others when I can. In the year 2019, I was a breast cancer model, recommended by my radiation team. Again, it's all because of God!

I didn't have any lumps, so you do not have to have a lump, and that's because mammogram exams are important.

Young ladies (any age), ask your doctor to test you for genetic trait if it runs in your family. Most importantly, men... Men can get breast cancer also, so it's important that you get tested.

This is my testimony, and I pray that this encourages all to not wait and get tested before it's too late.

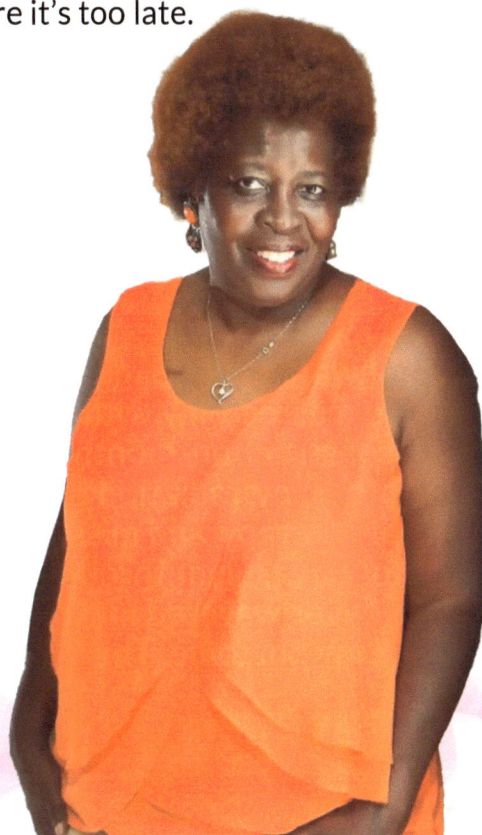

Ramonia Jackson Jenkins

As I think about my experience with cancer, I often say that I do not have a story to share. Well, in hindsight, my story is one of faith and survival.

When I got the diagnosis of breast cancer, I already knew my outcome. My faith was strong; and God had already revealed the pathway that I needed to take for my complete healing.

God never brings you to a situation or allows a test without already providing provisions to get you through. Though my journey and tests were quick and painless, my life's essence, trials and tribulations, had already prepared me to stand upon my faith and to abide with the Holy Spirit. For it was already revealed that I would be victorious over cancer.

My pathway included me having a double mastectomy with breast reconstruction, months of chemotherapy, radiation therapy, hormonal therapy, and missing time from work. As I went through these stages, I never wavered in my faith or doubted my outcome. The scripture speaks of having faith as a mustard seed and being able to move mountains. I used this scripture to remind me of the greatness of God and His ability

While it could be difficult at times to see and find the road through the trial called cancer - there is no right, correct, or proper pathway that we all must follow. Our survival rest within the particular journey that God has ordained though our faithfulness. I say, no matter the trial, be faithful in knowing that God has already made provisions for you. For now, unto Him who is able to do exceedingly abundantly above all that we ask or think, according to the power that works in us, stay faithful, be blessed.

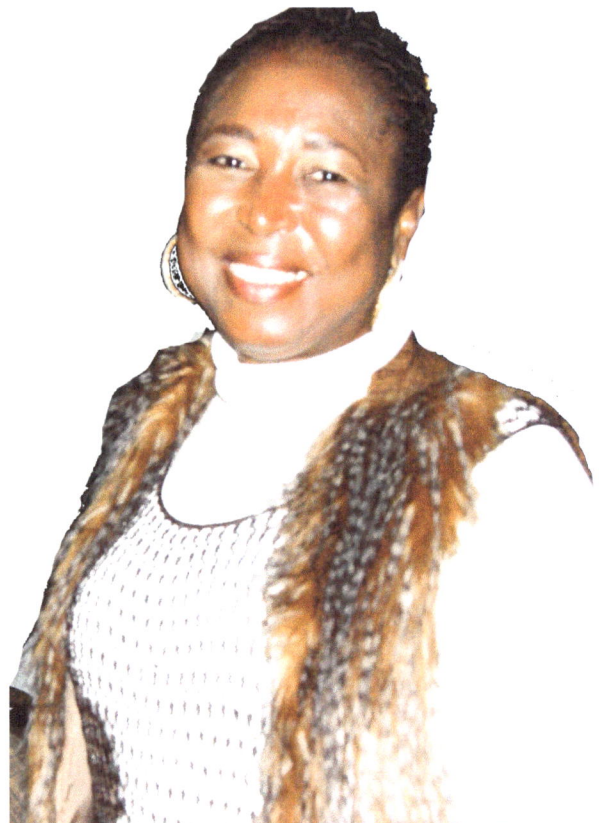

Talmadge Scott

I became a member of June Warriors through The Rule basketball team. While playing, I found out that Donald Price's mother was diagnosed with cancer along with his wife, Demetris Price. My mother, Naomi Katie Scott, also passed away from complications of breast cancer. So, I wanted to honor my mother and be a part of this special group of people that was helping fight this deadly disease. I asked how I could help in any way. Just tell me what you need me to do. So, I became a volunteer for the June Warriors, and I enjoy every opportunity to go out and support the cause. I cannot even imagine not doing my small part to fight alongside the June Warriors. This has become a family affair with my wife, daughter, and mother-in-law. We all support the fight.

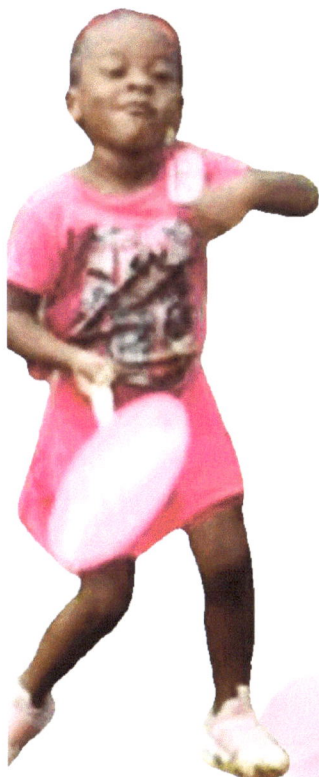

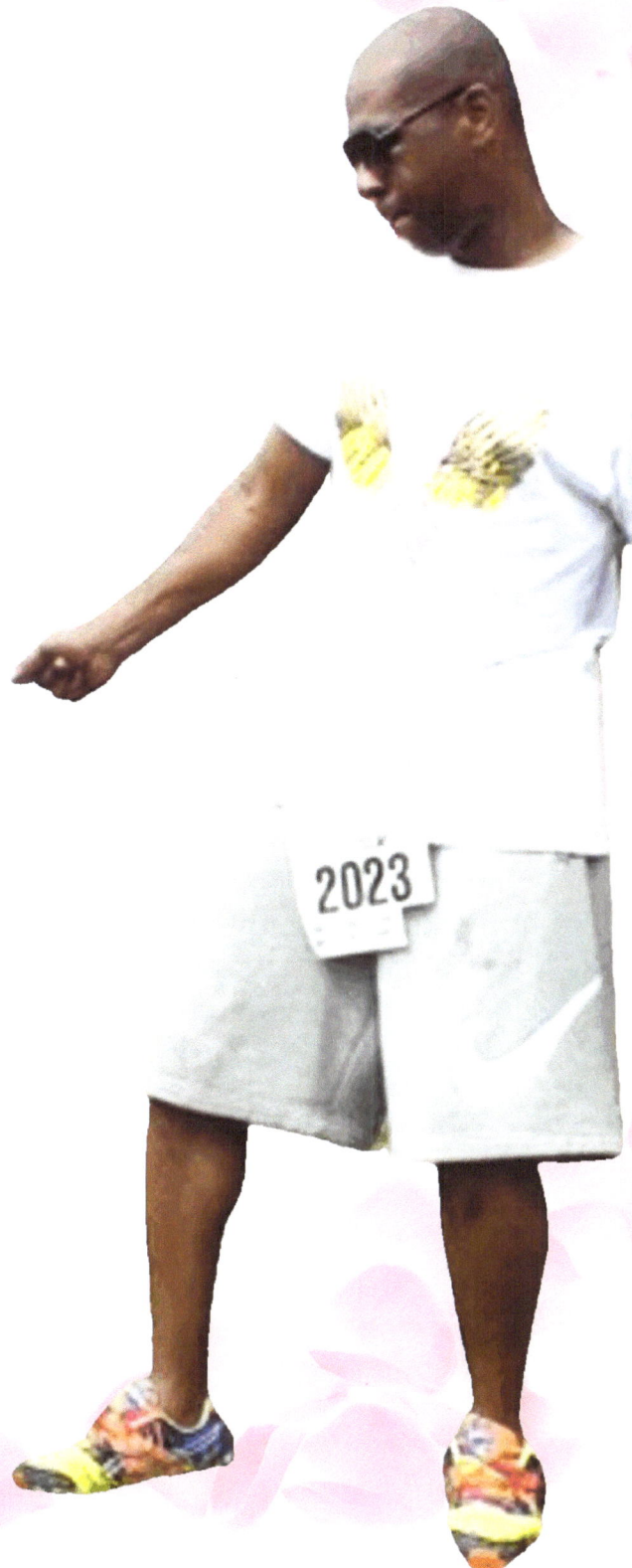

Ivory Haley Jr

and encouragement of family and friends. Even when the battle is lost, I see that my efforts at finding a cure is not in vain. Science and technology are changing each day to help find a cure. My prayer is that with my help, I may see the day when there is a cure for cancer.

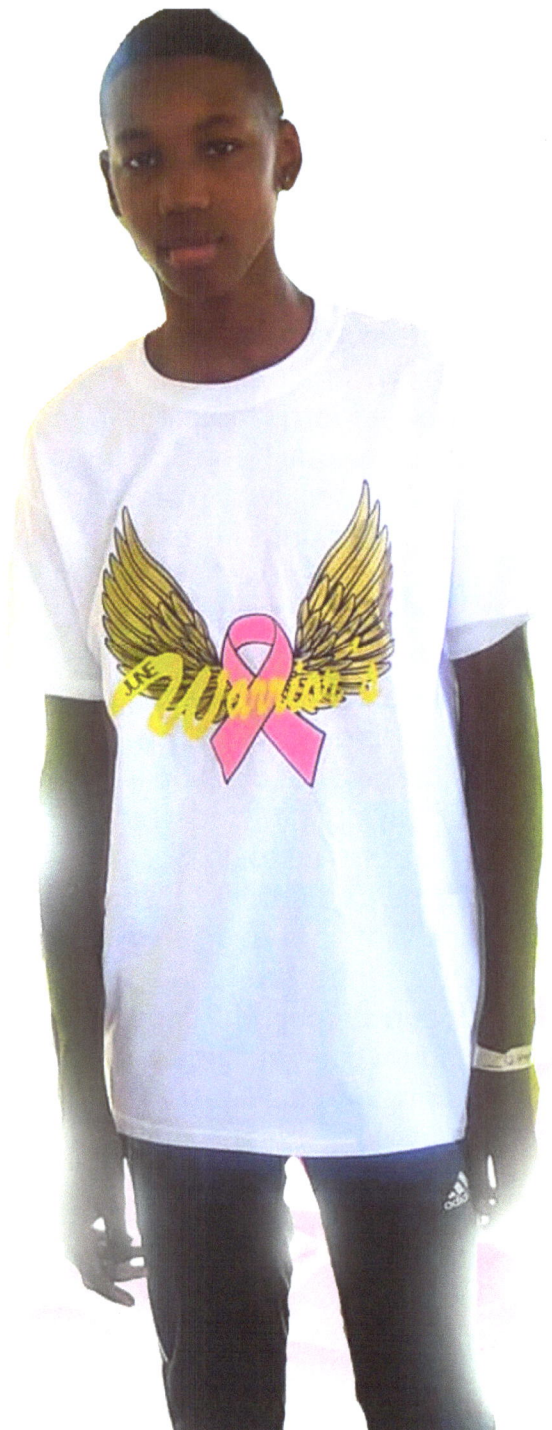

I have been involved with June Warriors as a boy up to I became a young man. I started by helping my dad grill oysters at the annual cancer walk in honor of his friend's mom, Mrs. June. At that time, Da Rule basketball team members helped to organize the food and activities at the cancer walk. A few years later, the June Warriors committee was formed. I continued participating in the walk, grilled oysters and began helping to set up and break down at fundraisers' events. By the time I graduated from high school, I received an award for having more than 100 hours of service time, thanks to my volunteering efforts with June Warriors over the years. The June Warriors committee even honored me with the Strong Man Award. June Warriors and their friends became my village, and they have inspired and enlightened me throughout my life.

At first, I thought when someone was diagnosed with cancer, death was imminent. After being involved with June Warriors, I see that is not often the case. My experience with June Warriors over the years has given me hope that cancer can be beaten with the support

Devin Price

Devin M. Price is the youngest son of Demetris & Donald P. Price Jr., the grandson of Selina F. Horton & of the late Donald P. Price Sr. & June Marie

Price McCarty. June Marie Price McCarthy was a 15-year Breast Cancer Survivor who lost her final battle against Breast Cancer in 2012. Demetris & Donald Price formed a committee named June Warriors and continued the team along with friends and family.

Their organization was formed through the love of friends and survivors. Every day from the day my grandmother was diagnosed, I have advocated the promise and, with the help and support of friends and family, has fundraised events all over the city. Being at a young age and witnessing what cancer can do on one's livelihood can change the way you think throughout your years. I have joined The Academia Society, Incorporated, to bring further knowledge to my community.

This is so that young adults like me can understand we are not alone in this world. If you do not know an answer, don't be scared to ask or reach out to seek the answer. I pledge to bring more knowledge to breast cancer to 18 to 24 years old young African American men so that they can understand and have the knowledge that young men can get cancer and, most of them all, Breast Cancer.

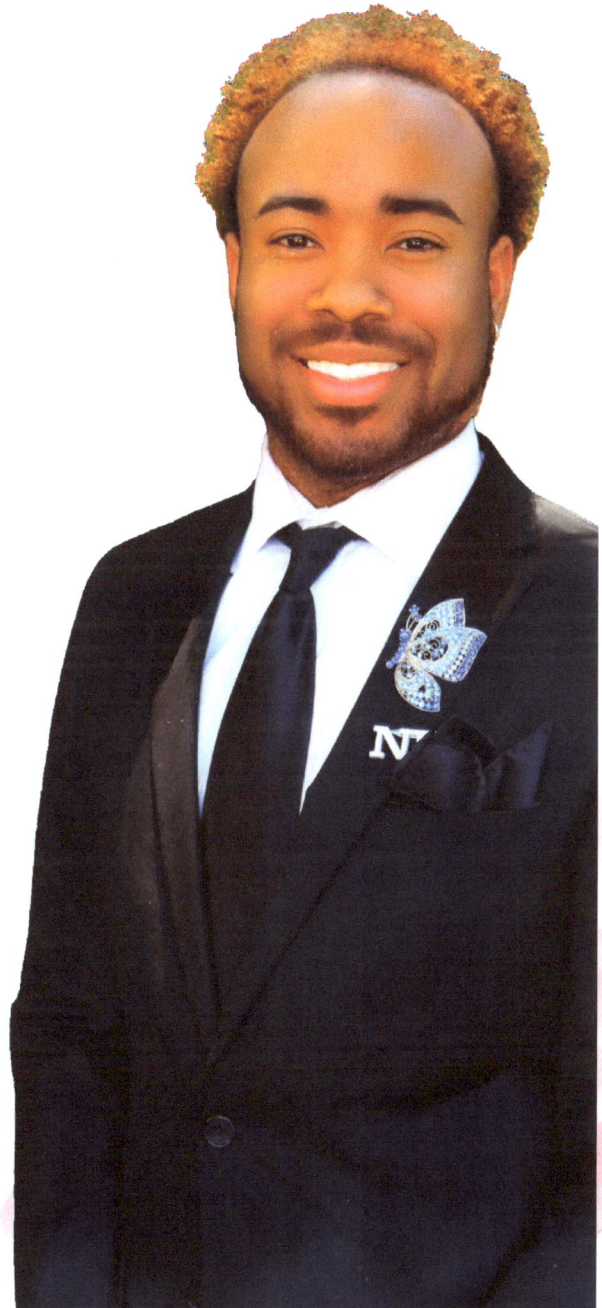

Eric Augustine Jr

My name is Eric Maurice Augustine Jr. son of Donald and Demetris Price. I started with the Warriors when my grandmother, June McCarty was diagnosed with cancer, and I still advocate for the cure today. It was hard growing up seeing someone you love in pain and there's nothing you can do about it but pray and be there to comfort them. Through the eyes of a child, this is devastating, and extremely hard to understand. I had so many questions and no answers.

They don't ask the kids how they feel, but we see and have many questions. I do whatever is needed to help my mom and dad from setting up for the events to fundraising. My immediate family comes out and support. Even though my fiancé, Adrianna Ferrell, has a cancer team, her family and friends joined in with June Warriors each year to help fight cancer. From a child, now a man, I understand the importance of getting tested and having good health. Learning along the way to be able to pass the information on about awareness. Men can get cancer too and it runs in our family. I have a son, Eric III and he's been advocating with us since he was born. Family is everything, having a strong support group is key and keeping faith is important. I was taught to never give up. June Warriors is a group of individuals who are more than friends. We are family.

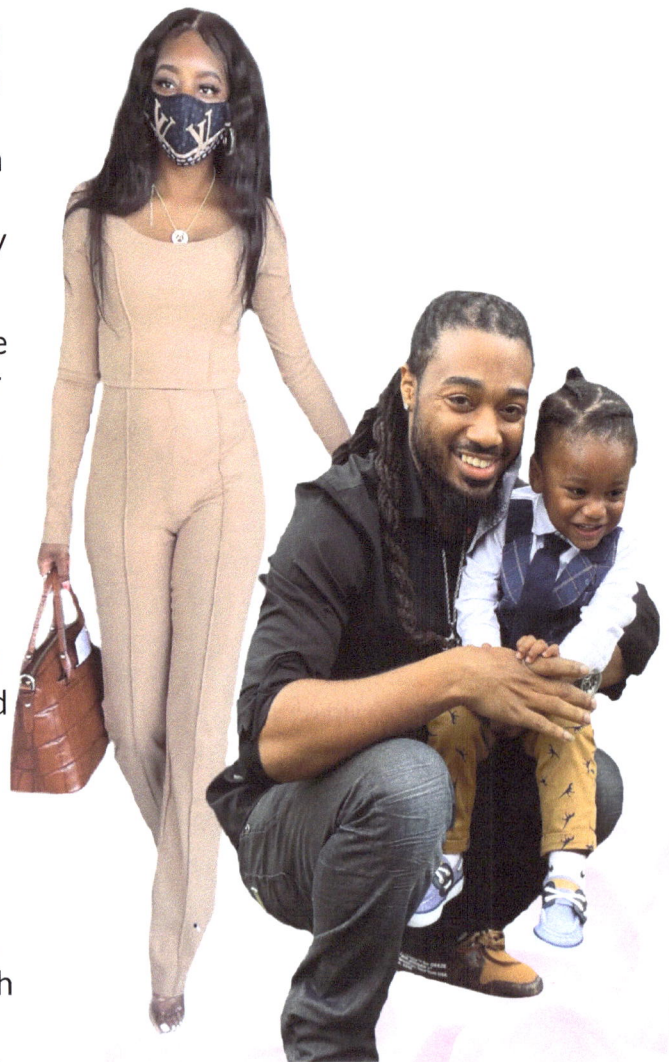

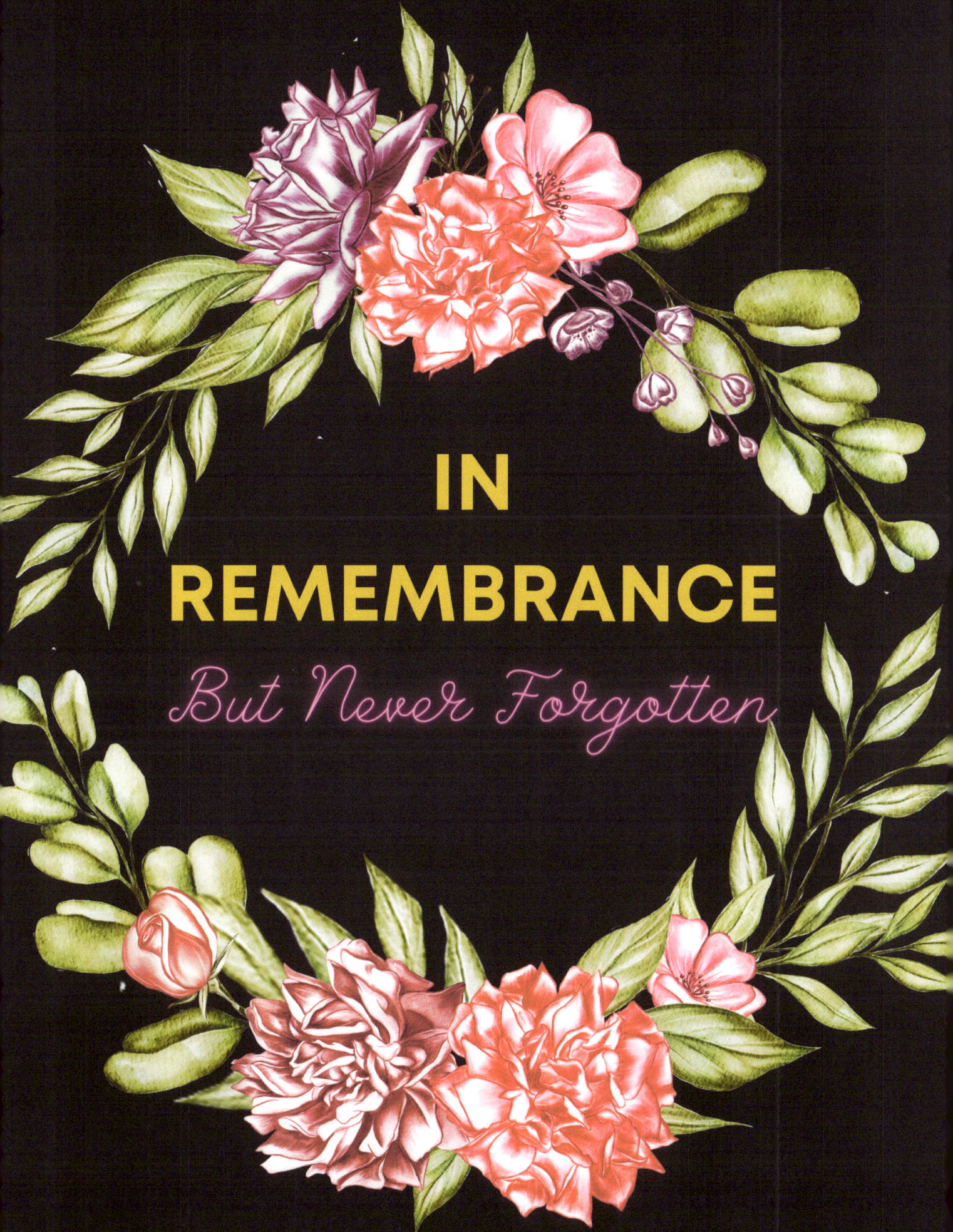

IN REMEMBRANCE

But Never Forgotten

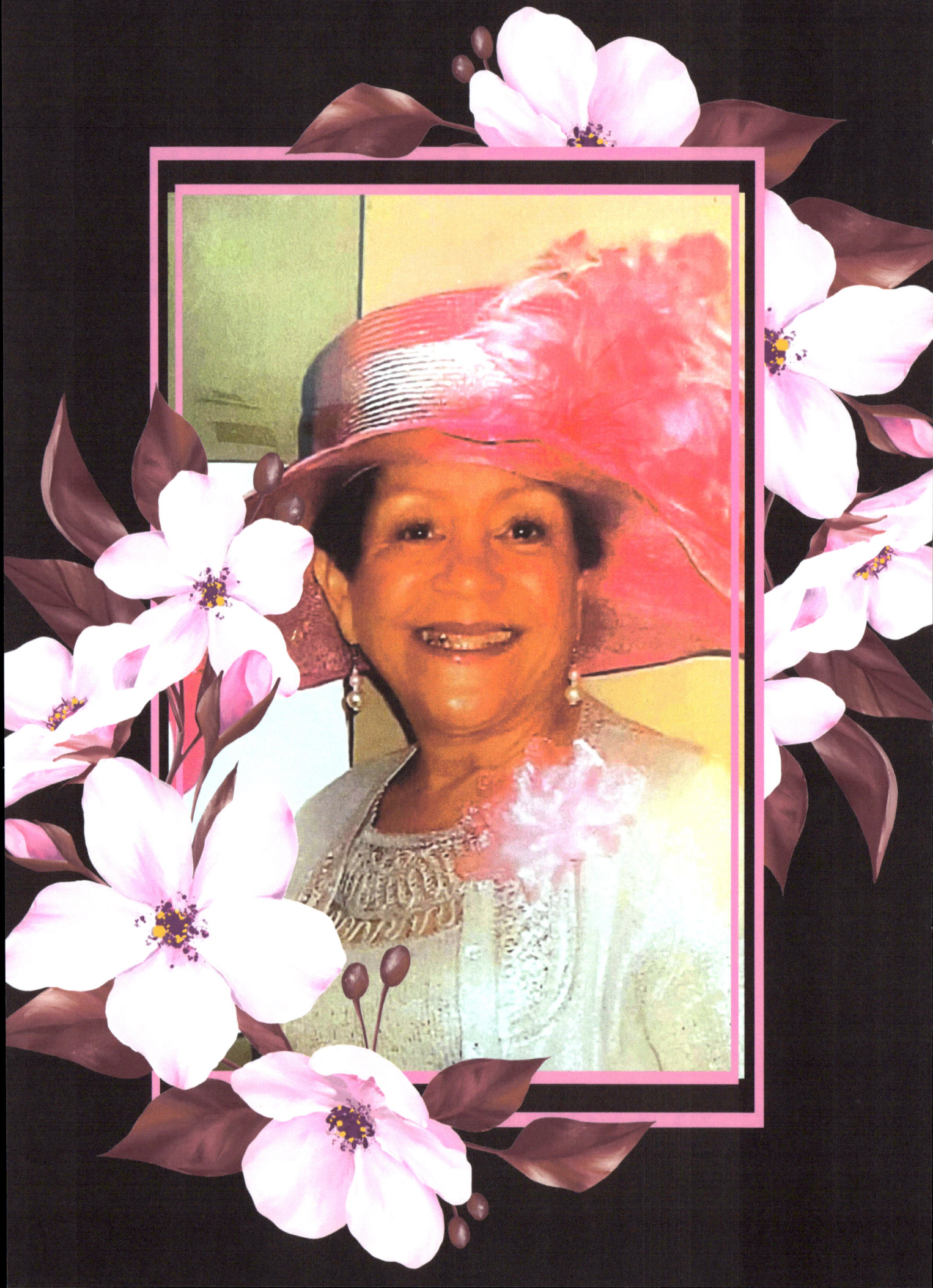

June Marie Wallace Price McCarty

Sept. 01, 1950 – April 03, 2011

A breast cancer diagnosis in 1994 motivated June to become a tireless, committed advocate for breast cancer education and awareness; a caring, loyal friend and supporter of survivors; and a dedicated advocate for the vision of Susan G. Komen for the Cure to end breast cancer forever. She championed educational projects including bringing Komen on the Go to New Orleans, raced in DC, in the National Race and advocated at Lobby Day. Her Second diagnosis only served to strengthen her resolve to work harder.

June Marie Wallace Price McCarty, a retired Chevron, USA worker of 28 years, entered eternal rest on Sunday, April 3, 2011. The loving wife of Moss McCarty. Jr. the mother of Donald Phillip Price, Jr. (Demetris). Sister of Stanley J. (Claranecia), Carmen A., Gail R., Bruce M. (the late Rose), Matthew (Terry), and Anthony (Odelia) Wallace. She is also survived by 3 grandchildren: Eric M. Augustine, Donald P. Price III and Devin M. Price, along with a host of nieces, nephews, other relatives, and friends.

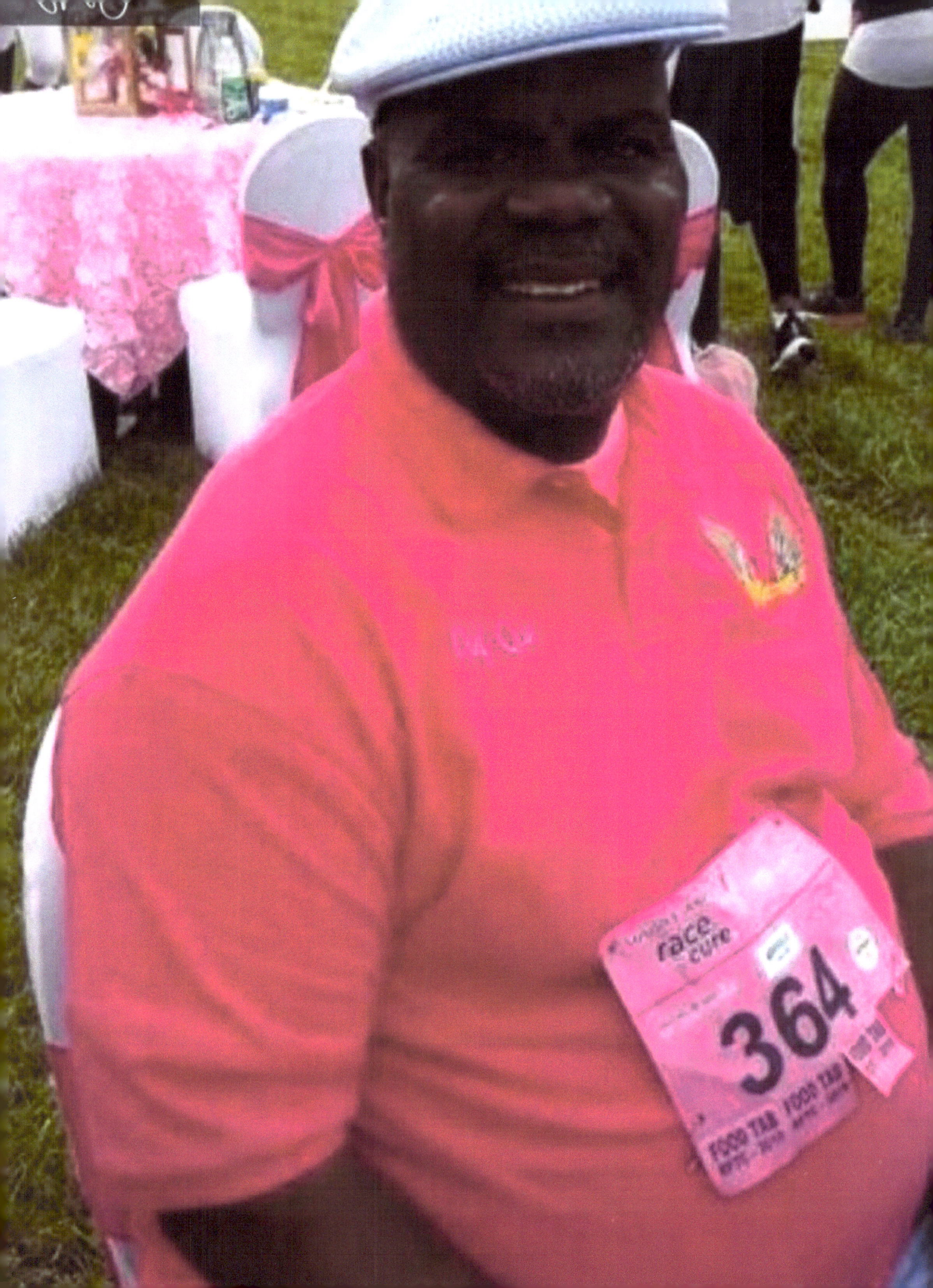

race for the cure

364

FOOD TAB

Quinton Irvine Jason

April 6, 1965 – Sept. 26, 2020

My name is Quinton Irvin Jason. I would like to thank God for his mercy and grace. I was a two-time stage four cancer survivor. After finding out I had colon cancer, it was very scary at first, but I was ready for the challenge. God is so good. He places people in your life to help you, and to help keep the faith and hope alive. One of my high school friends had stage four cancer. I admired how he was so positive about it. He is eight years cancer free. He helped to motivate me and inspired me to go to the gym and workout. We both do this five days a week. I believe this person was placed in my life by God to help me push on. Kent Shelby always encourages me to workout hard and eat right. If I missed a workout, he would call to see if I was okay. Sometimes, when I was tired of my chemotherapy, I would pray to God for a good treatment.

I always stayed around positive people to keep me strong and motivated. Going into the final treatment was brutal, but I thank God, and I also thank my wife, Jackie Jason who is my strong arm. The lord God said, "*It is not good that the man should be alone; I will make him a helper fit for him.*" Genesis 2:18 That is my Jackie. She was there when I was about to give up. She held it up when I could not. That is what I mean when I say God puts people in position. All Glory be to God for saving me.

Now my goal is to help other cancer survivors. I have joined this incredible organization called June Warriors. The people in this organization have uplifted me on my good days as well as my bad. It is great that God has blessed me and placed me in a position to help other cancer survivors and those who are still suffering in the beginning stages.

Thank you, Heavenly Father in Jesus' name, Amen!

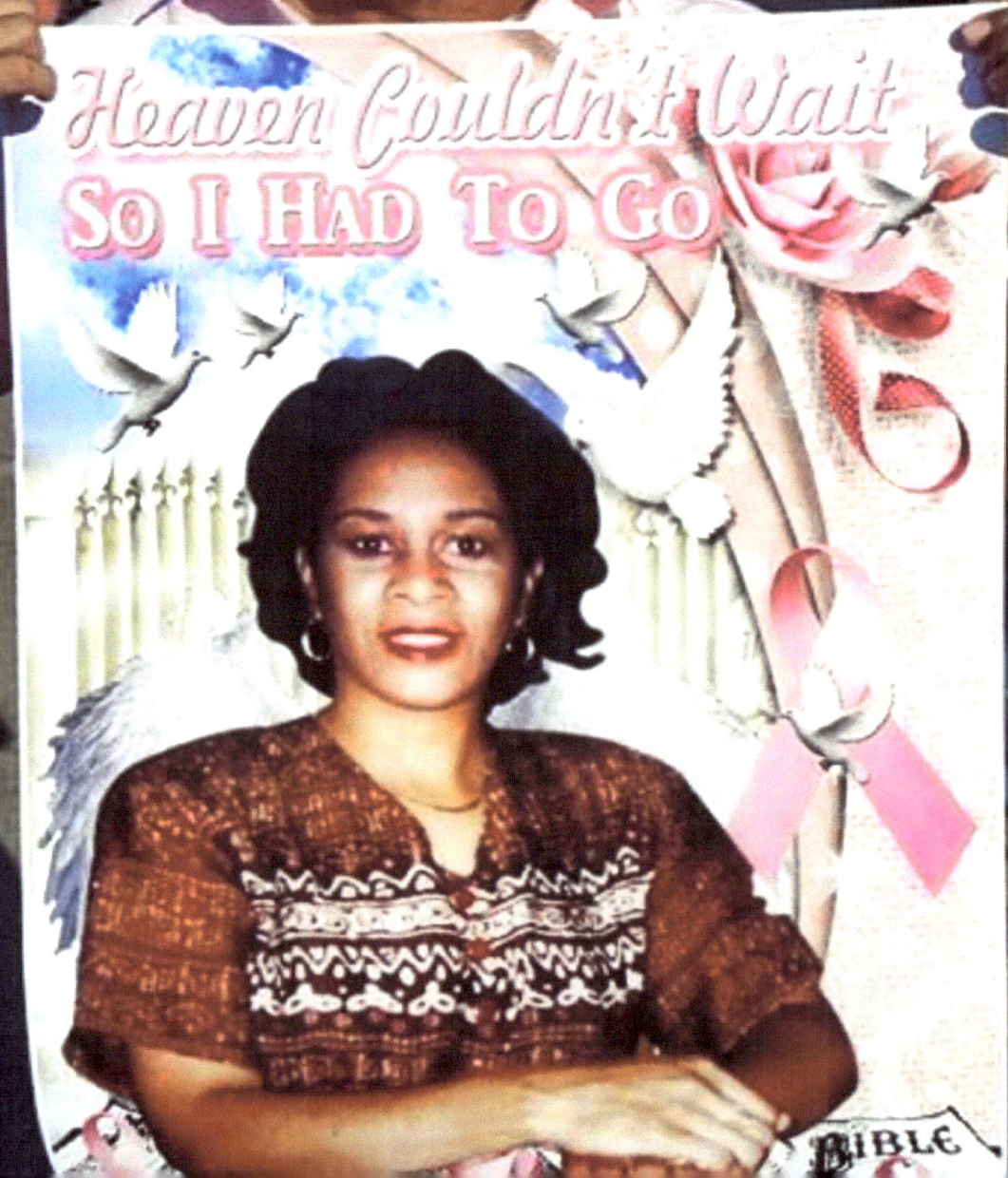

Heaven Couldn't Wait
So I Had To Go

BIBLE

Zenobia Williams Garcia

May 21 1961 – Dec. 29, 2009

Beloved wife of David Garcia went home to be with the Lord on Tuesday, December 29, 2009, at the age of 48. Mother of Danielle-Jariece (Jason) Seymore, Jacqueline-Nicole, Marianne-Elizabeth, and David-Christopher Garcia.

Zenobia had a beautiful spirit, and you would never see her without a smile, known as Zee by most. Zenobia fought a good fight. The battle was not hers; it was the Lord's. Loving mother and wife always had an encouraging word and a great sense of humor. True Warrior.

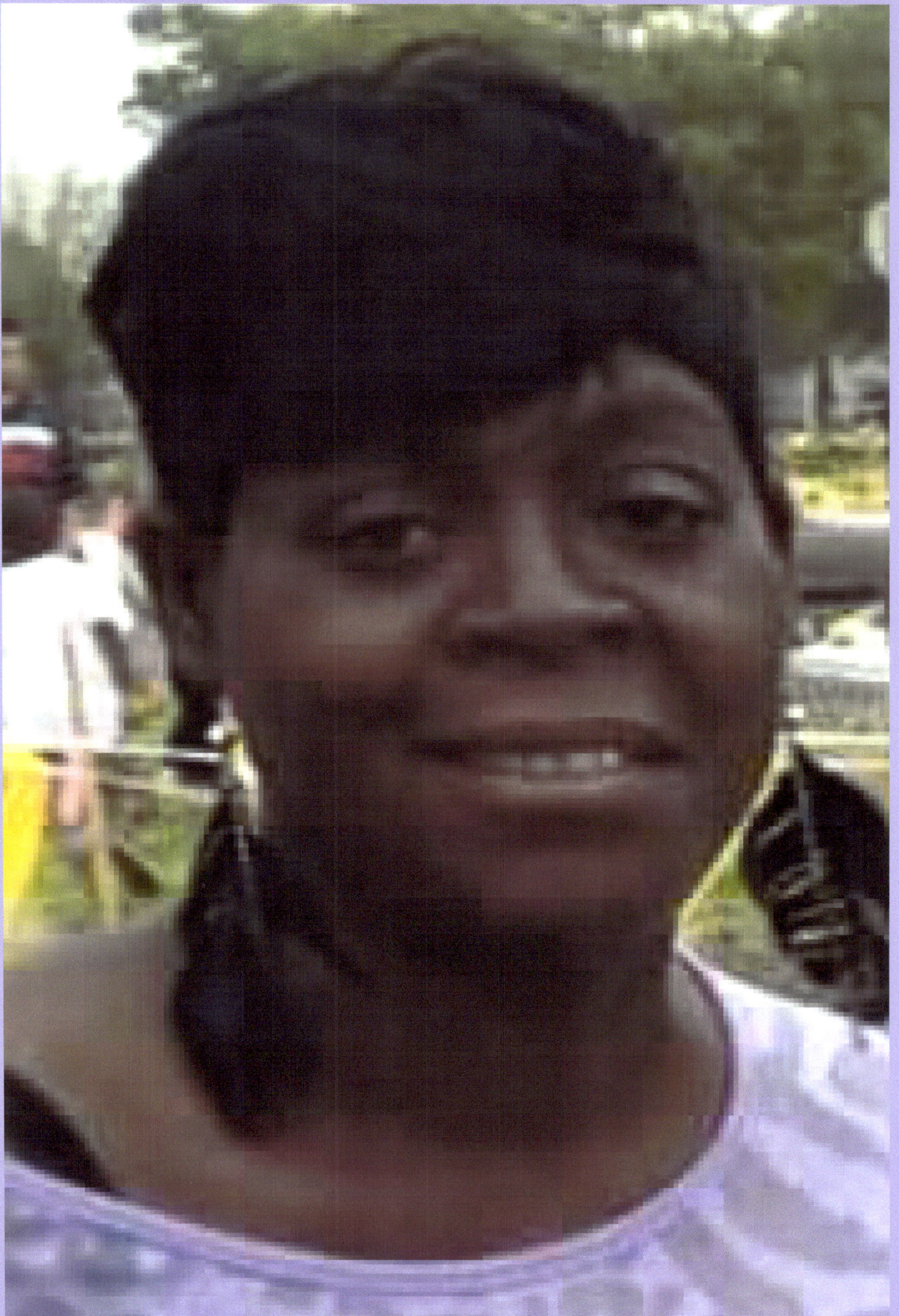

Tanya Rose

August 31, 1968 – Sept. 25, 2017

A daughter, wife, mother, grandmother, sibling, and friend. This is her legacy. Tanya Rose was happy, fun, loved to dance, and was ready for a good second line. She was a thoughtful and caring person. If you ever needed some place to lay your head, she would welcome you to her home. She always loved to entertain company and was well known. She was a great cook, you would never leave her house hungry, her food was finger licking good. She had her life ups and downs, but she took it all in stride, taking it one day at a time.

When she was diagnosed with cancer, she never wavered. She is one of our guardian angels sent from above. She is deeply missed. Her memories will continue to be with us forever until we meet again. Tanya Rose departed this life at Touro Hospital on September 25, 2017, at the age of 49. Beloved wife of the late Devin Mark Rose.

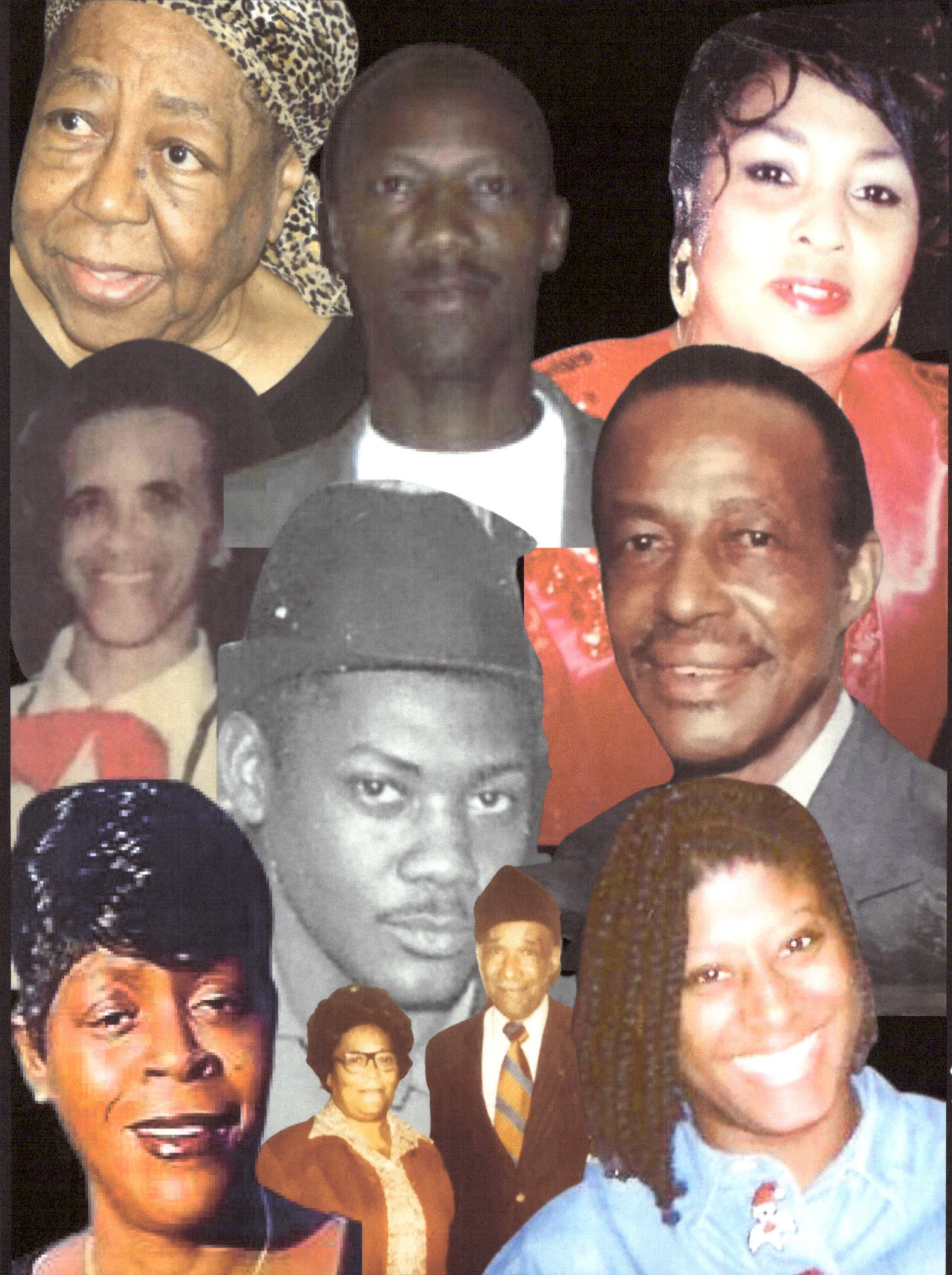

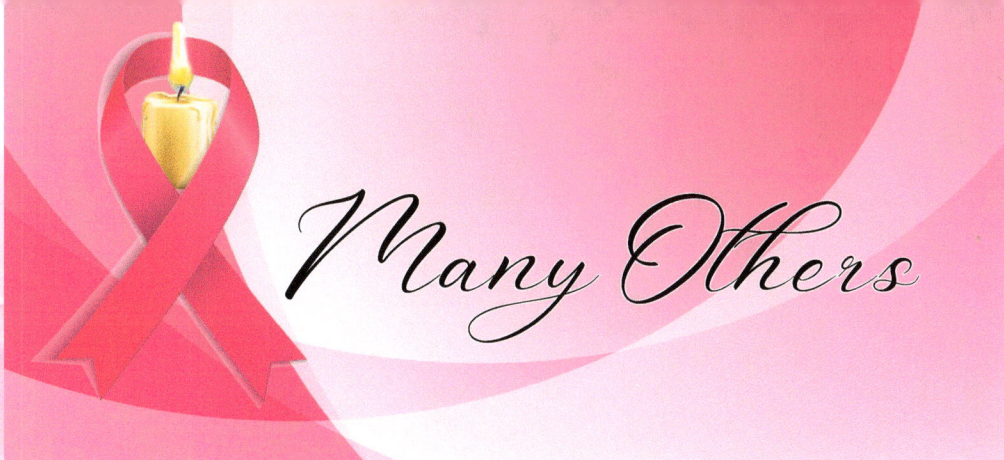

Many Others

Lester Jack Washington
Susan Marie Wallace Hunter
Donald Phillip Price
Rose Wallace
Francis Melson
Prince Bernard Melson
Naomi Katie Scott
Susie Jackson Legeaux
David Wilkerson I
Alvin Richards
Louise Cowart
Charlene Pratt
Billy Newell
Larry Phillips
August Richards
Marvel Richards
Edward Thompson

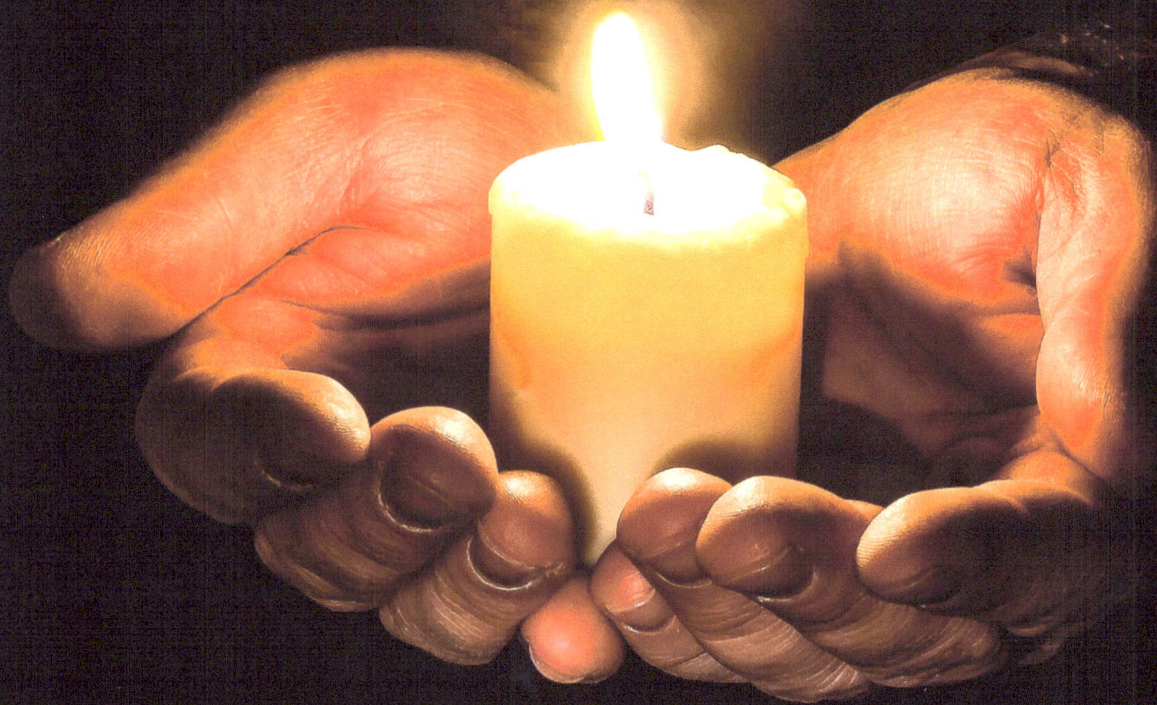

OUR LOVED ONES

THE TRUE WARRIOR

By: Donald P. Price III *"Cellophn"*

One may hear the word Warrior and think of the Battlefield,
but sometimes, those battlefields lie closer to home than you think,
not just out of the country.
These battles may lie within, mentally, physically, and spiritually.
You hear Warrior and you think of a soldier,
a person who's fighting for a cause.
But we have Warriors around us in many forms.
Our Mothers, Father, Sisters, and Brothers.
See, I'm here to tell you about the people
who've been fighting a battle
that seems never ending
but their souls aren't giving up on the war within.

Their light shines brightly in the face of each obstacle.
Not knowing which way it may take them,
but they're fighting to show their loved ones
that just because something doesn't work out in your favor
doesn't mean you should lose hope.
You see, these warriors are the foot soldiers
who carry the torch for the ones before
and the future warriors to come.

They carry that flame to let anyone,
and everyone knows that as long as you carry that flame,
you can light any path that seems to be closed or dark.
So, when someone asks me what makes someone a warrior,
I stare and I think about my grandmother,
still fighting even when she saw that the tunnel leads nowhere.
She wanted us to know that until you can't fight no more,
until that last breath is in you,
fight and keep hope in you.

See, the true warrior is the warrior who carries hope in their heart.
That hope touches and travels across the battlefield,
and that hope fills everyone that comes in contact with it.
That hope gives them the strength to fight harder,
to come back home.

The true warrior is one who carries wisdom,
compassion, understands pain, fears the battle,
but understands the war.
That warrior is the beacon of light, so I say,
"Shine on warrior, may your light lead us home".

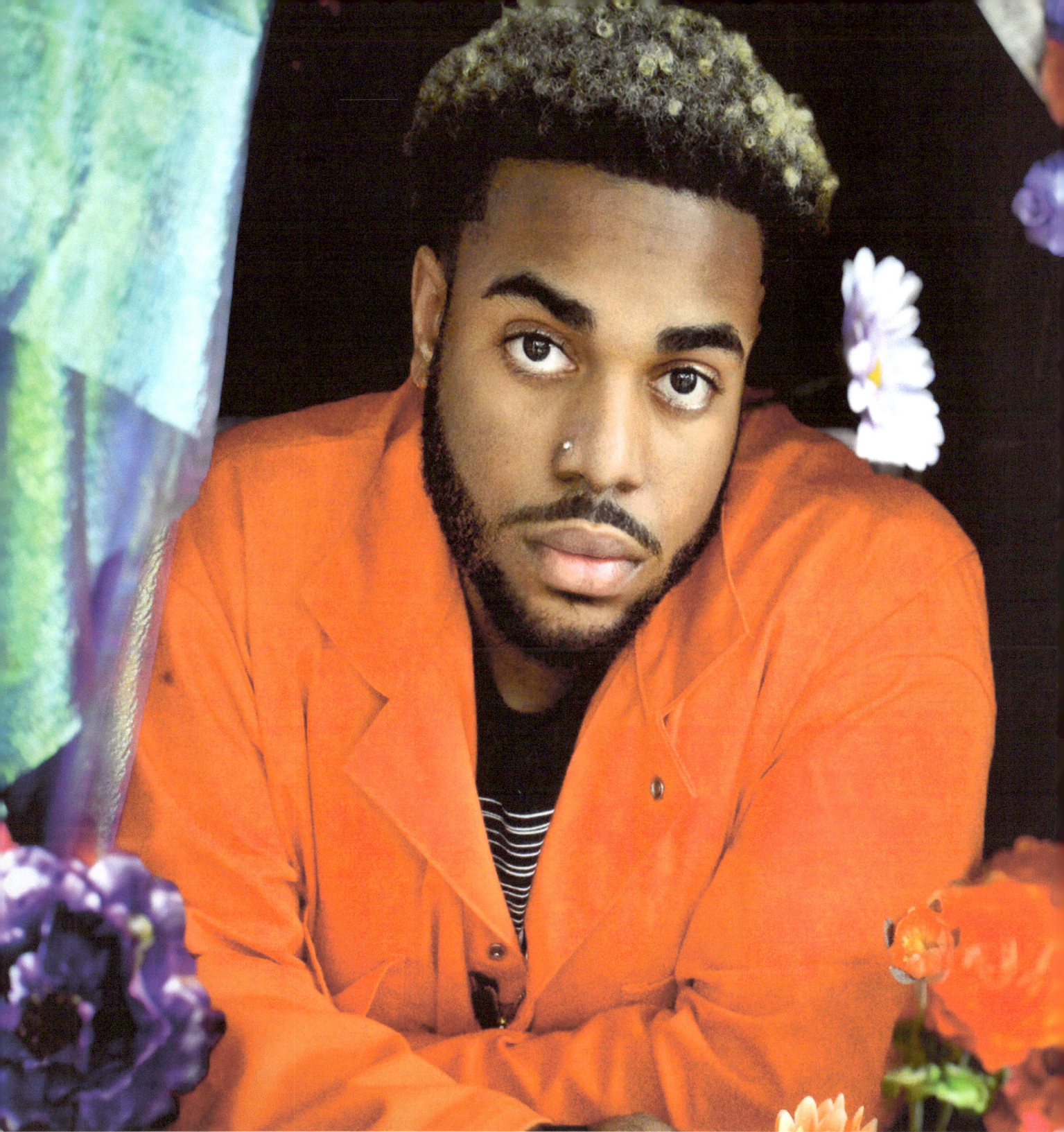

Donald Price JJJ "Cellophn"

Scan the QR code
to see the video
with the poem.

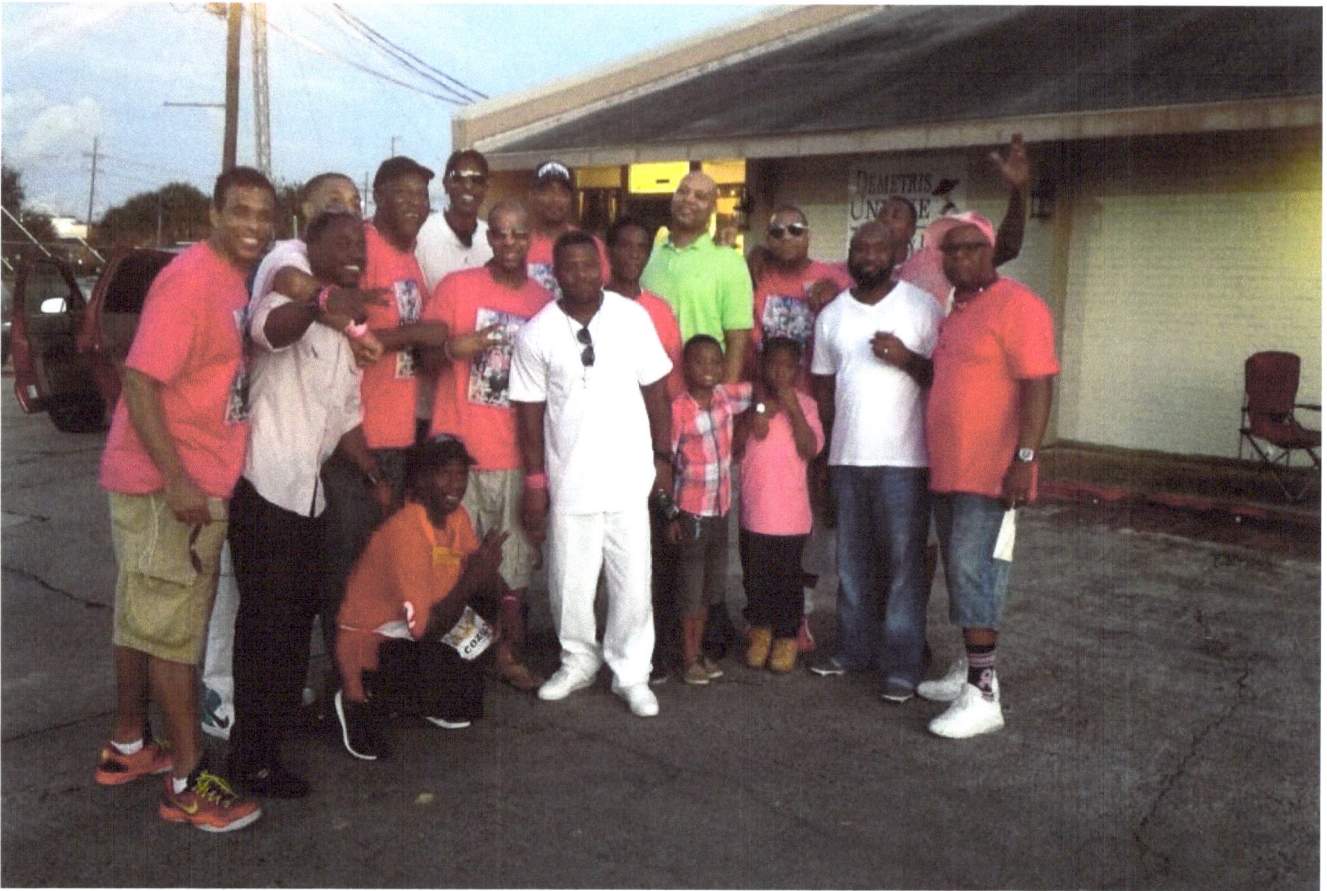

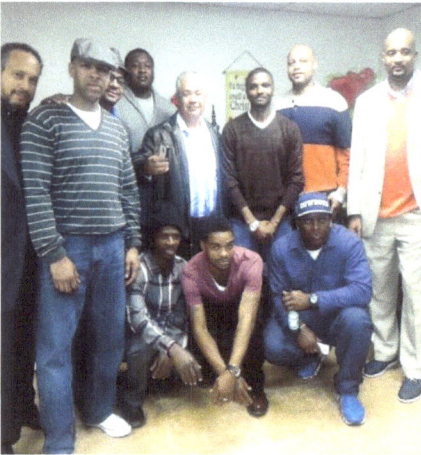

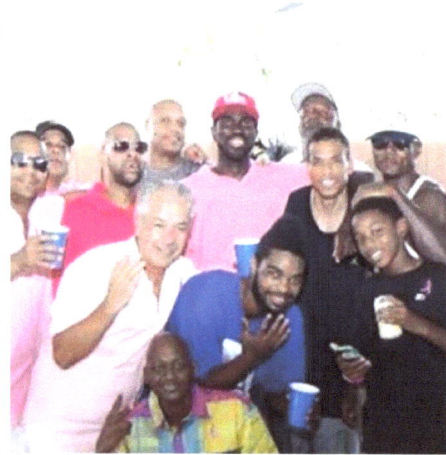

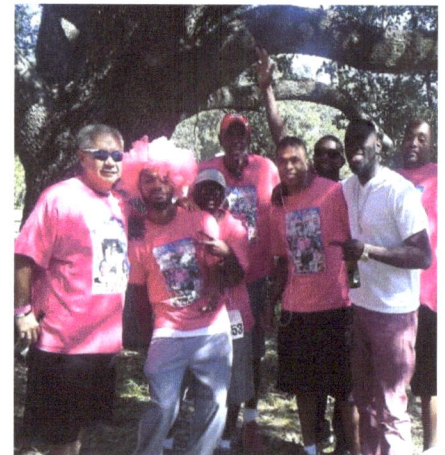

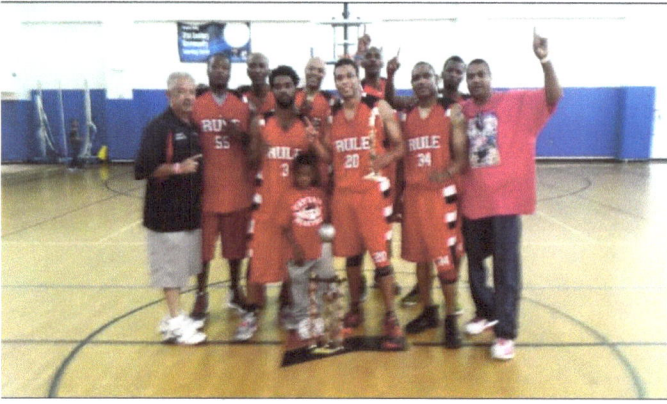

THE MEN

THE RULE

BASKETBALL TEAM

The men who supported the cause when I started.
Grateful for your unlimited support.

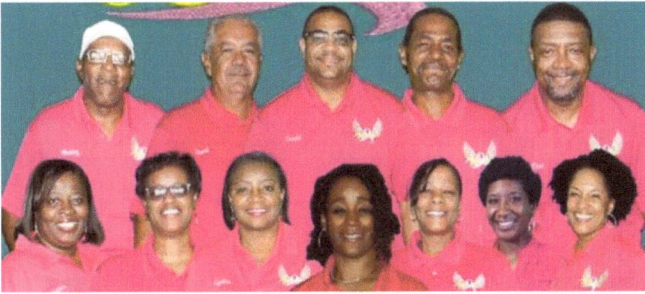

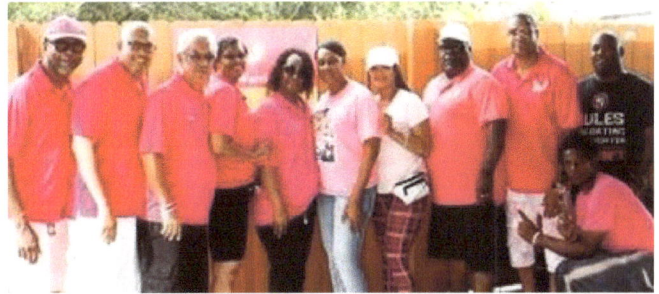

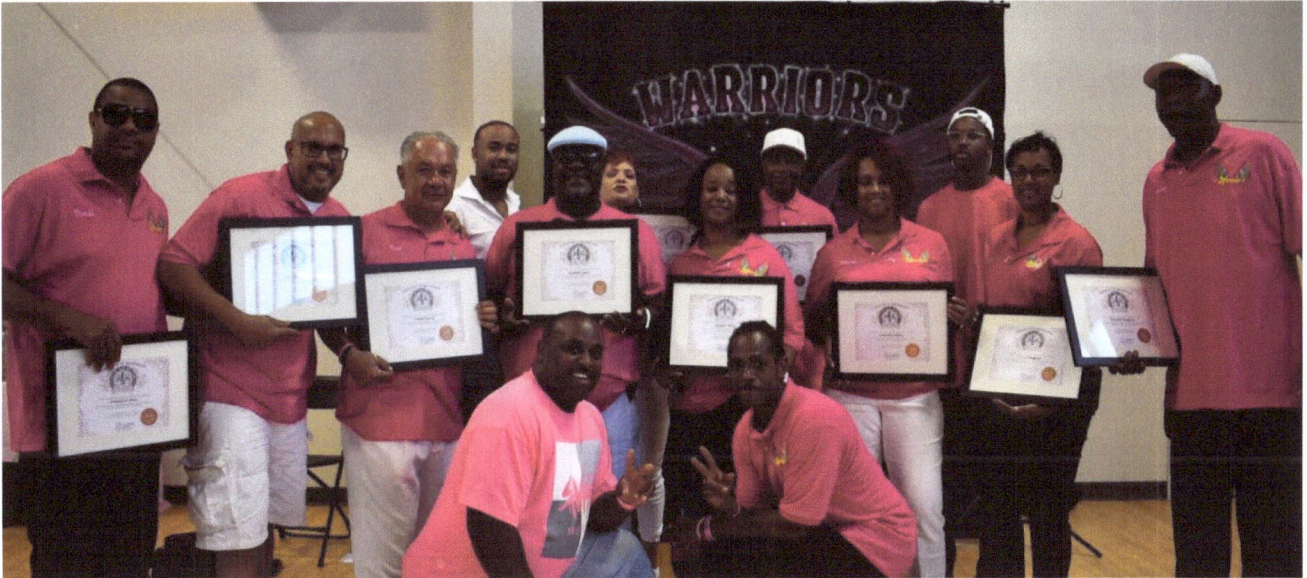

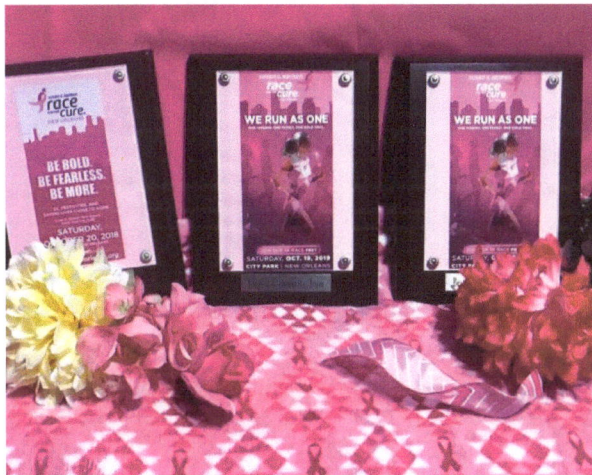

PAST

PRESENT

FUTURE COMMITTEE

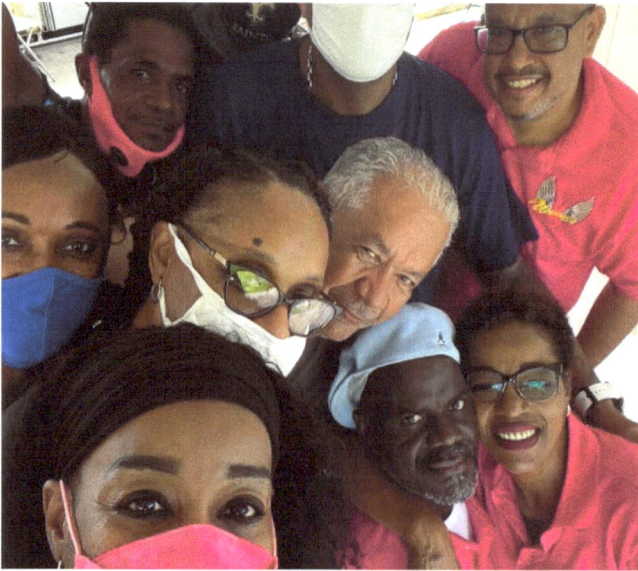

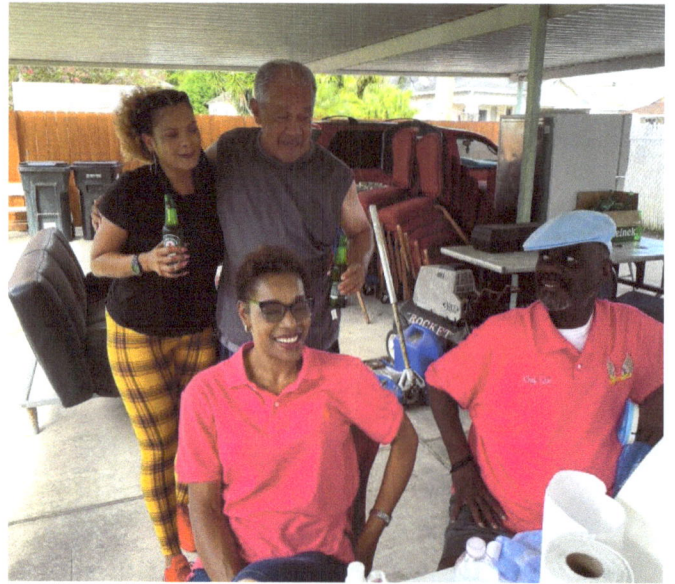

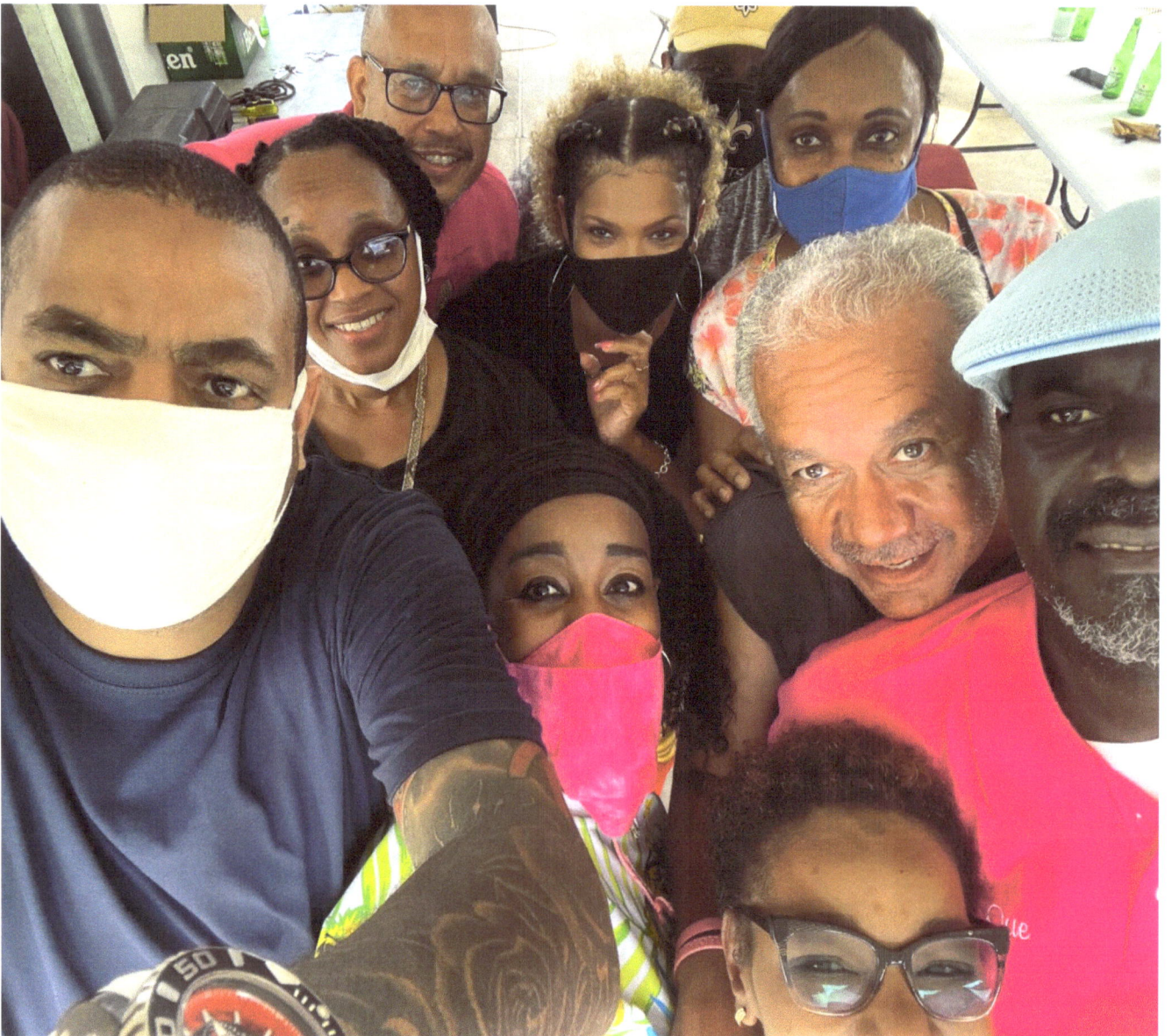

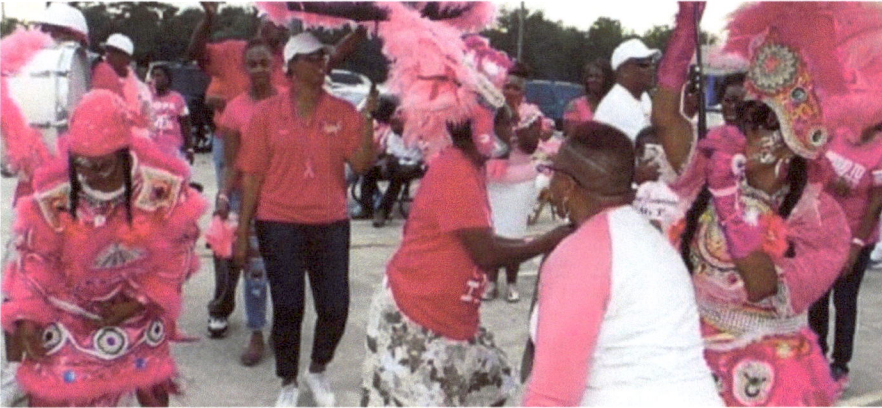

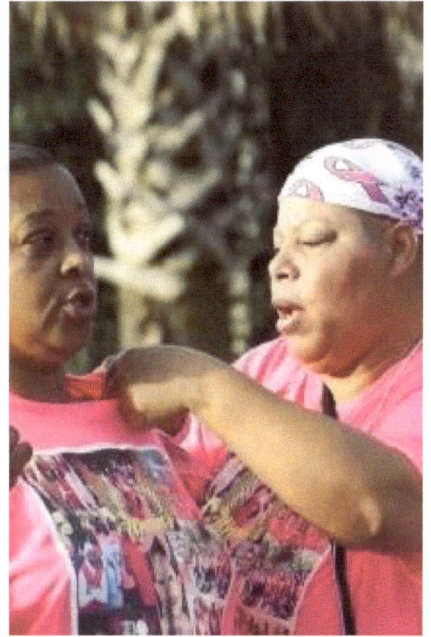

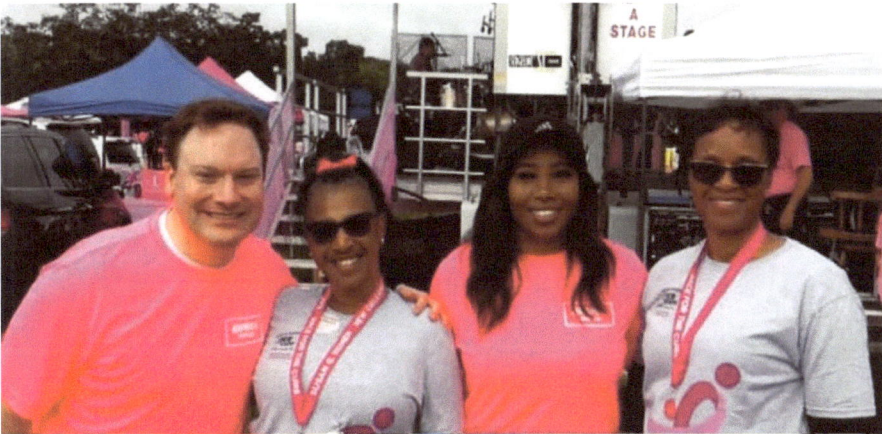

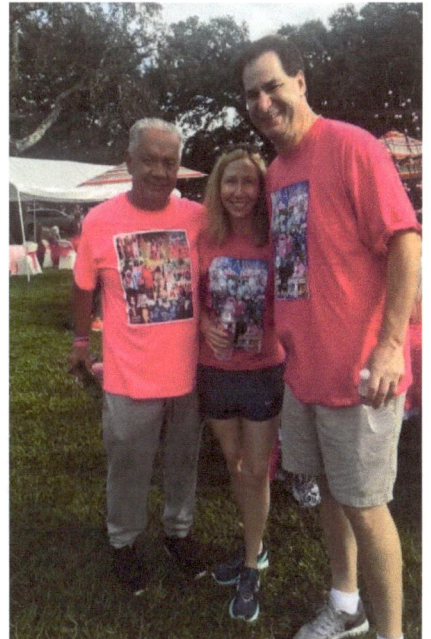

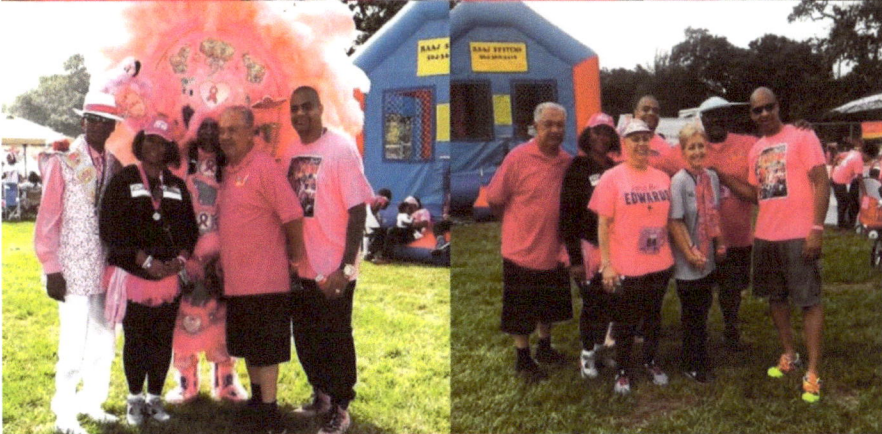

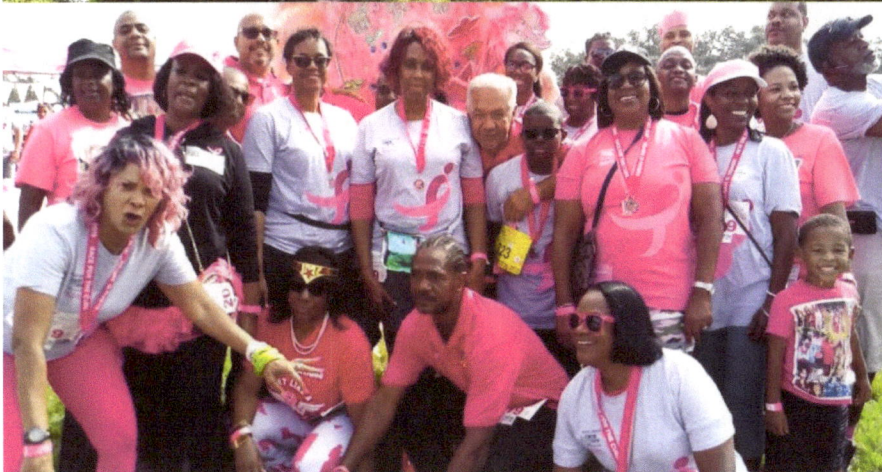

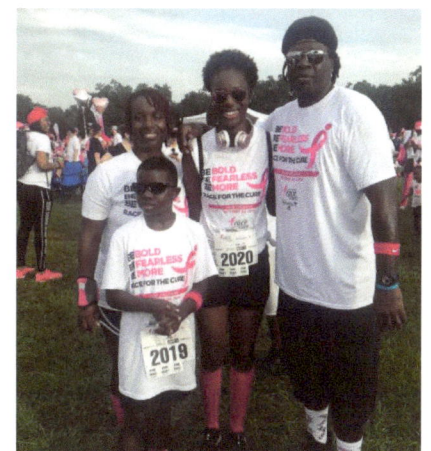

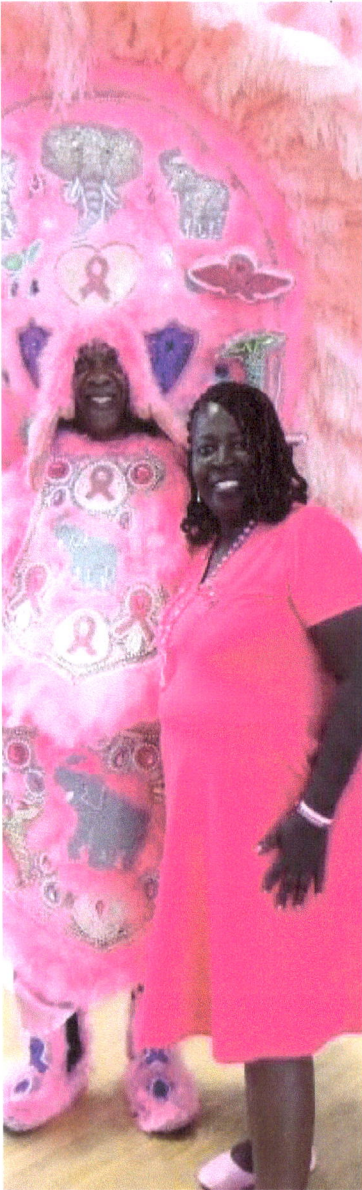

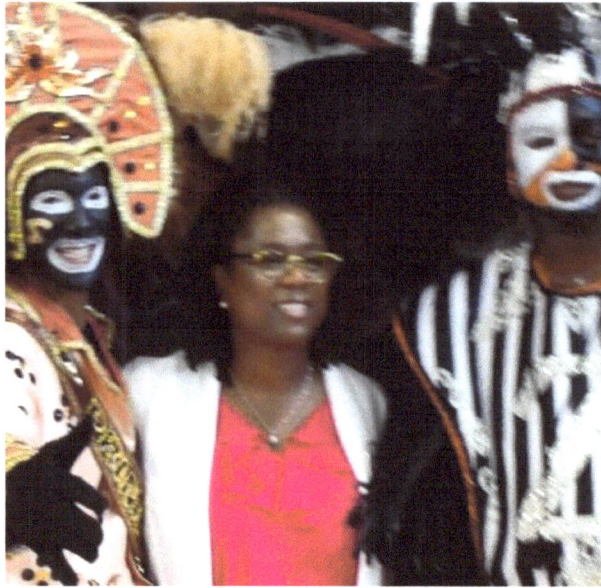

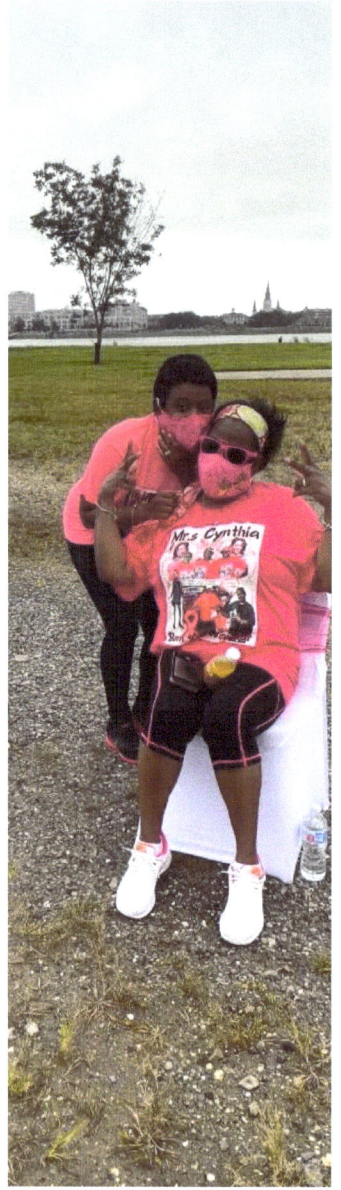

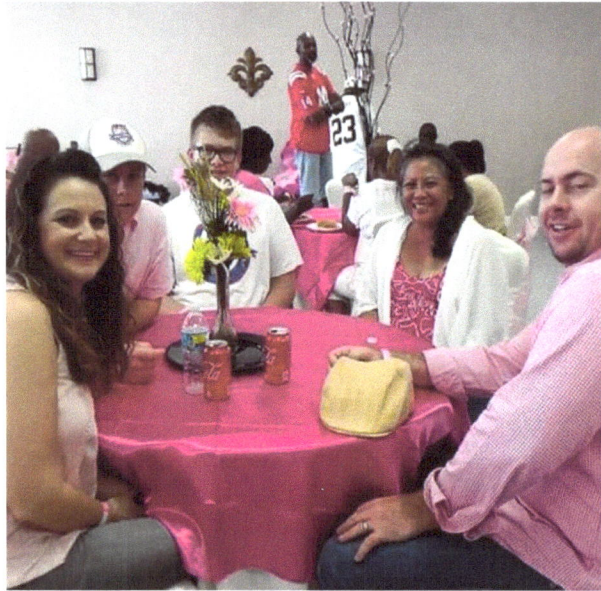

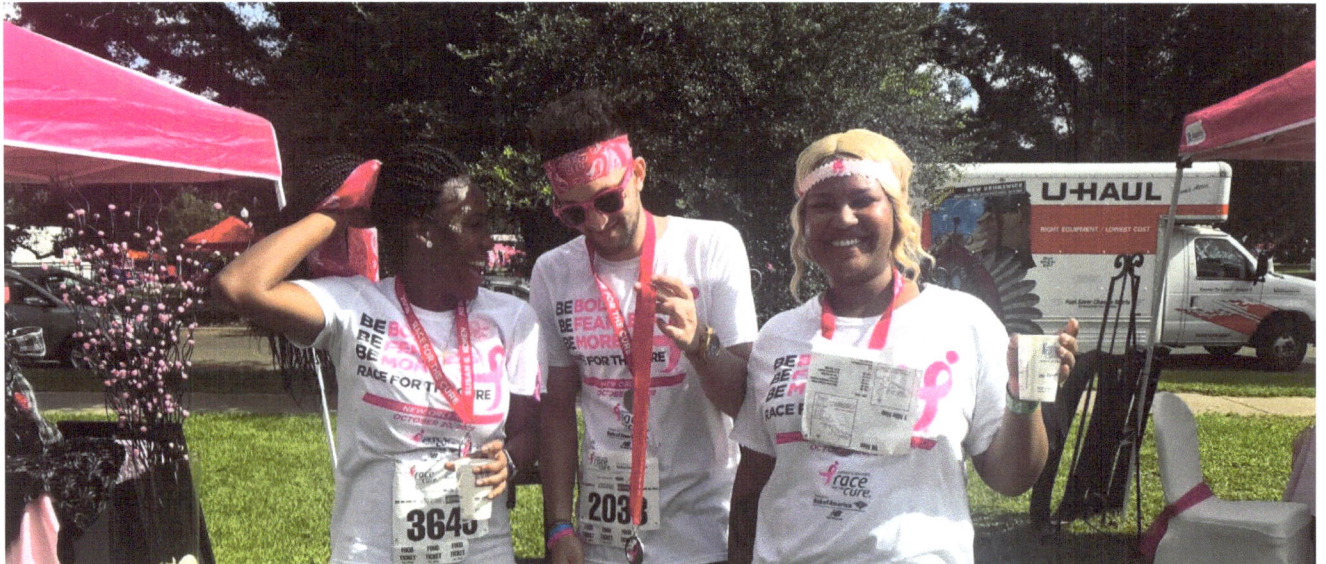

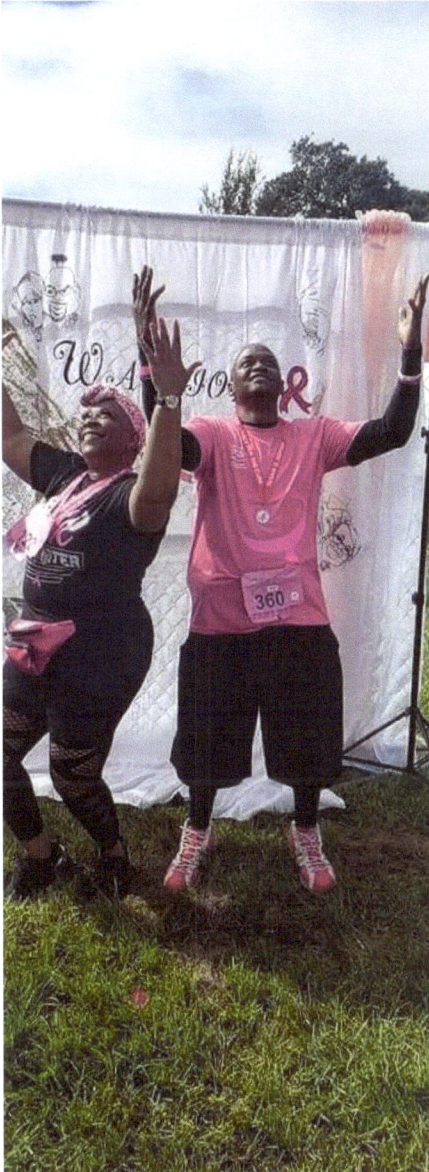

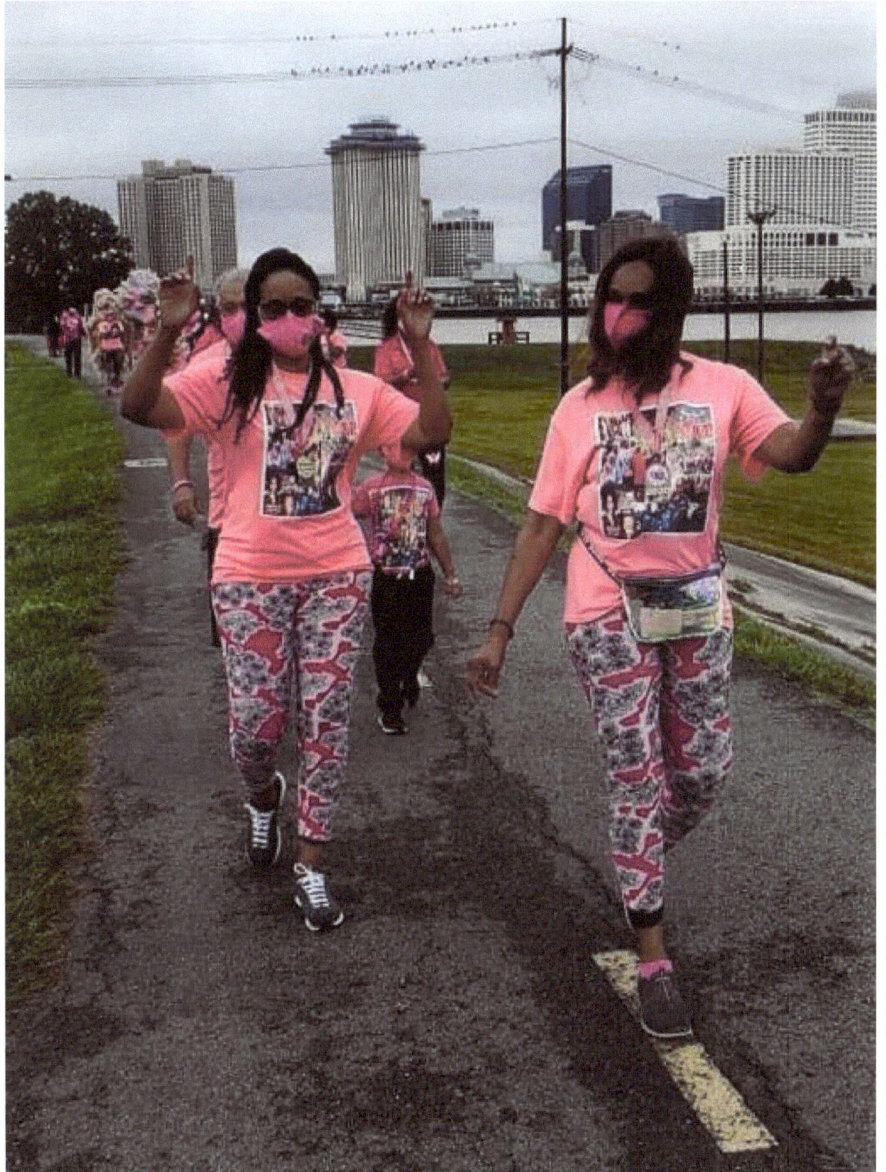

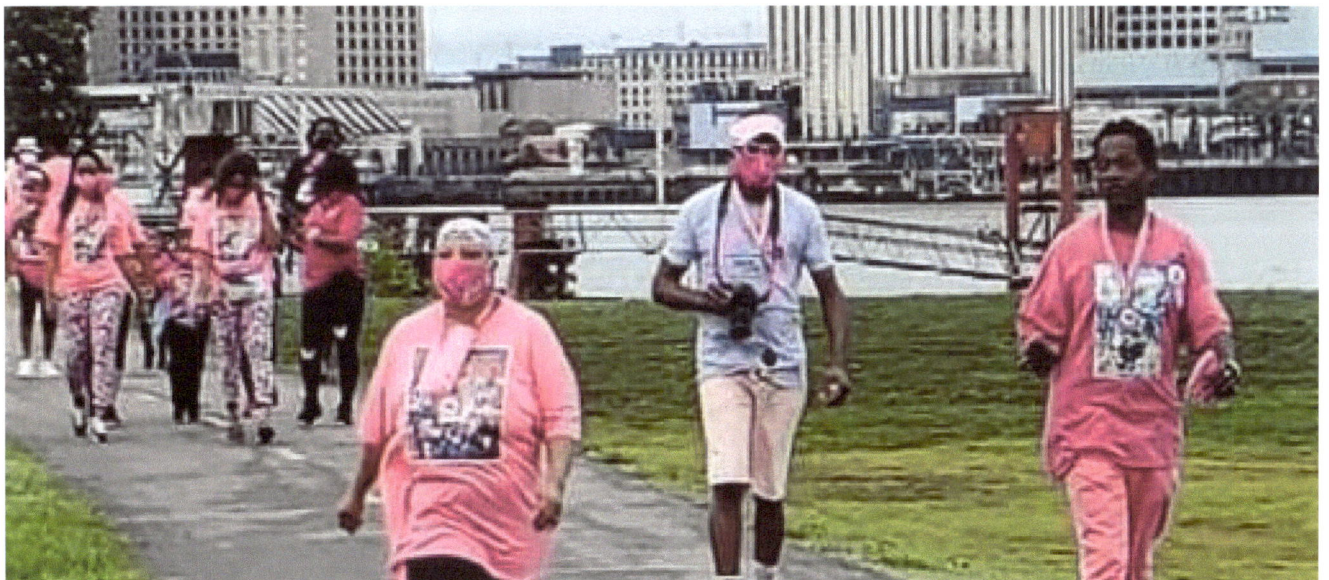

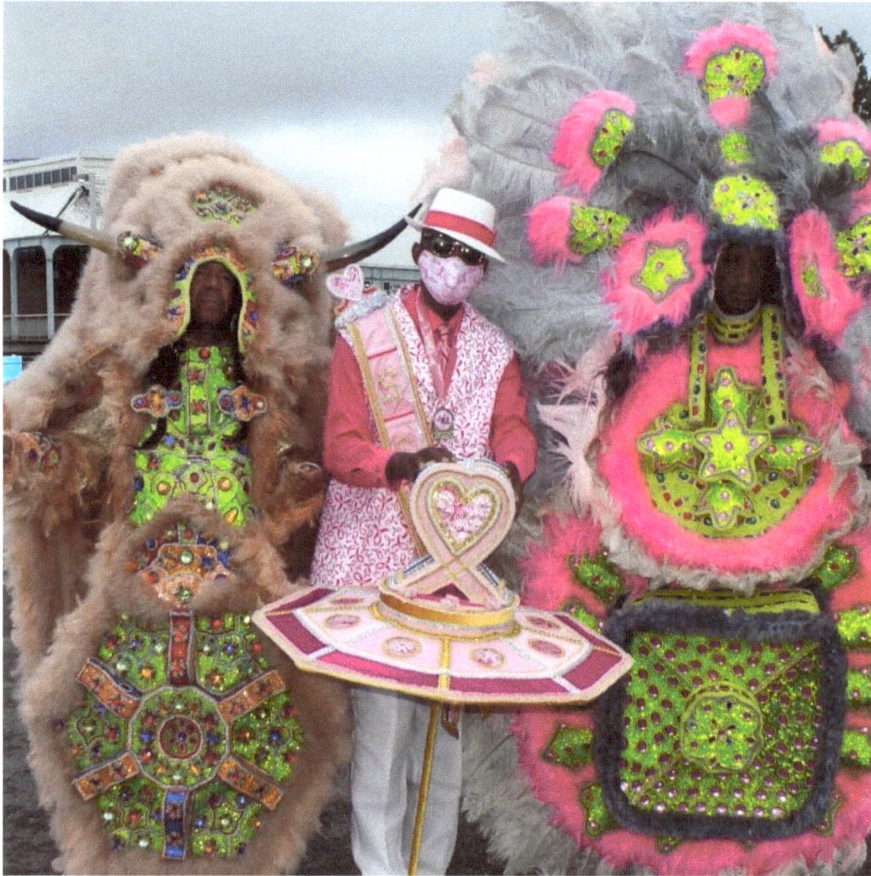

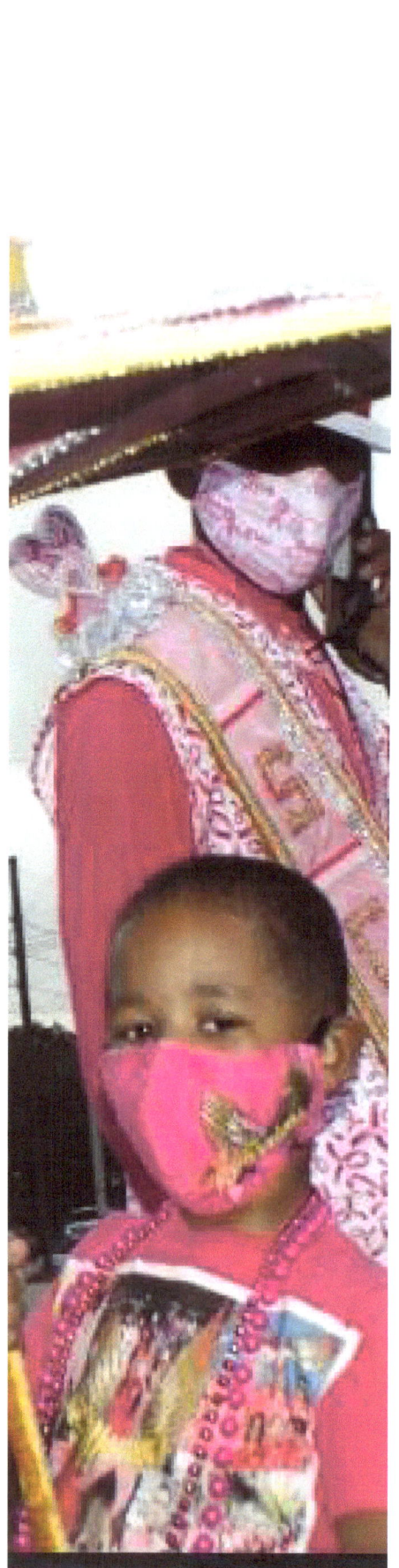

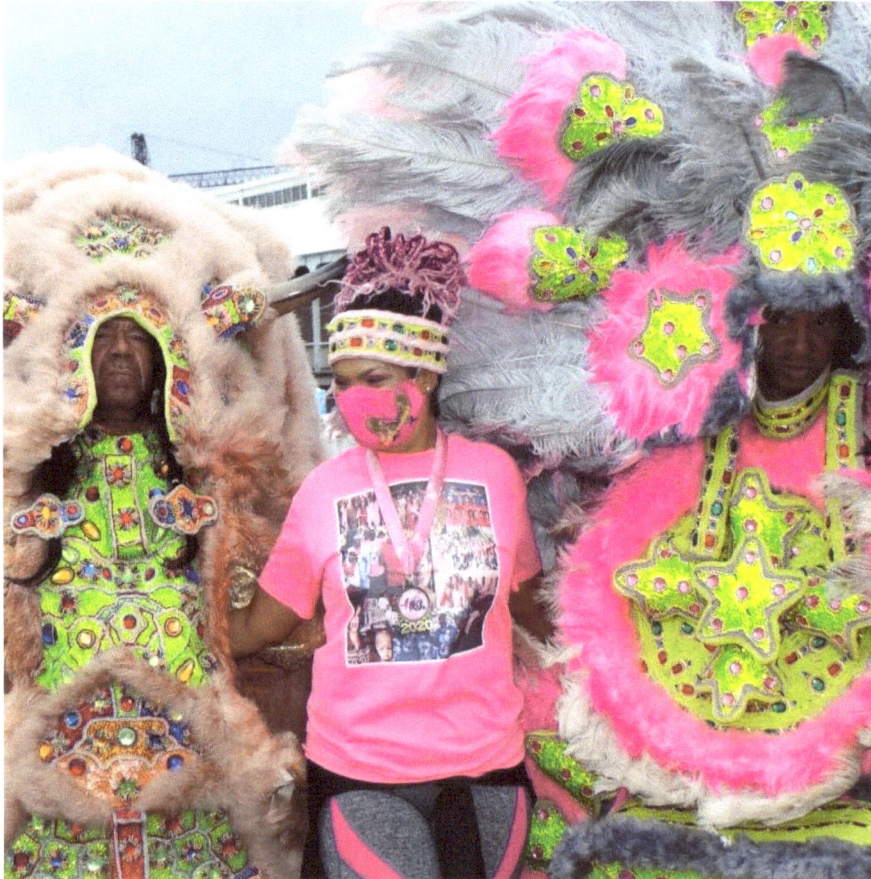

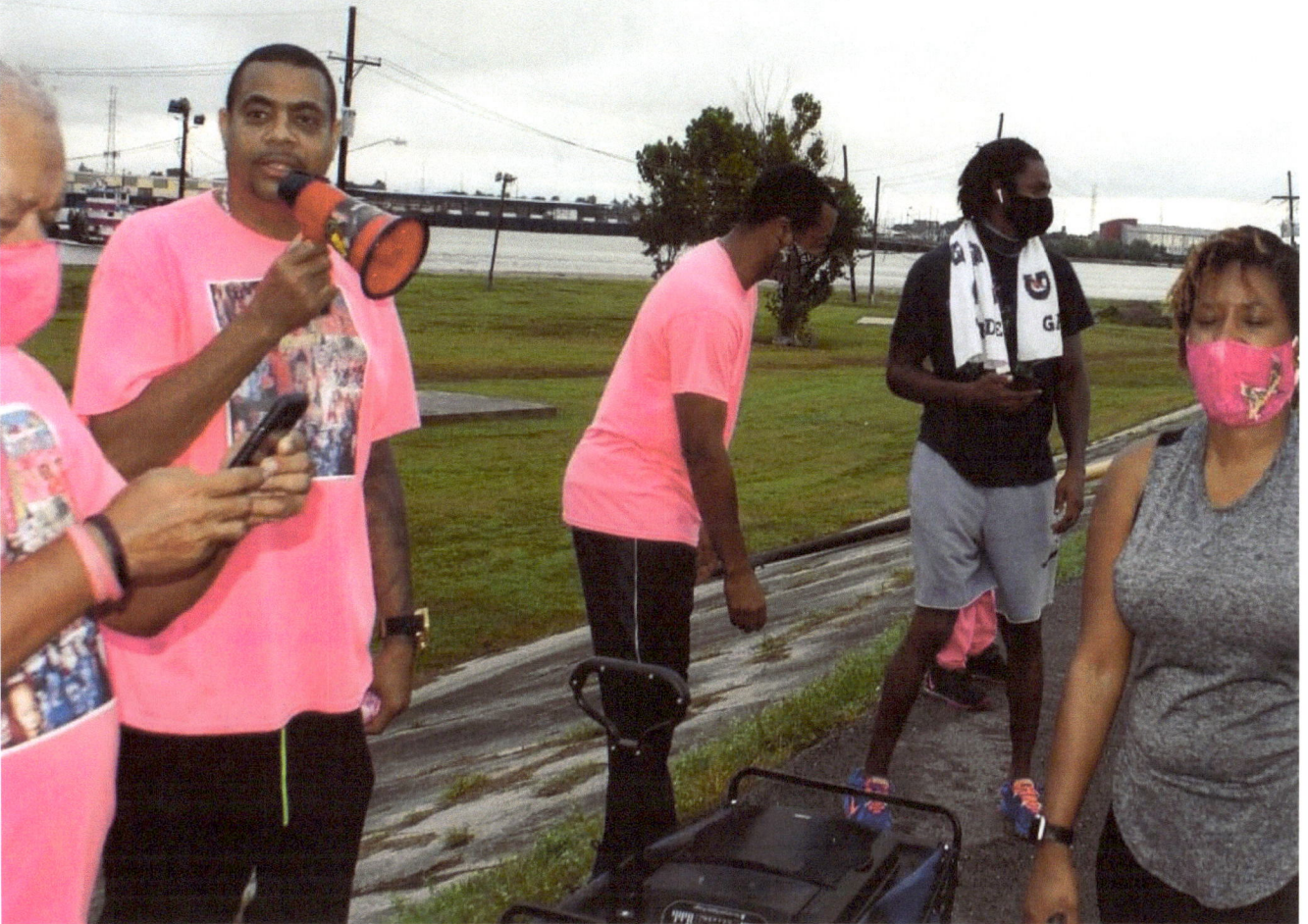

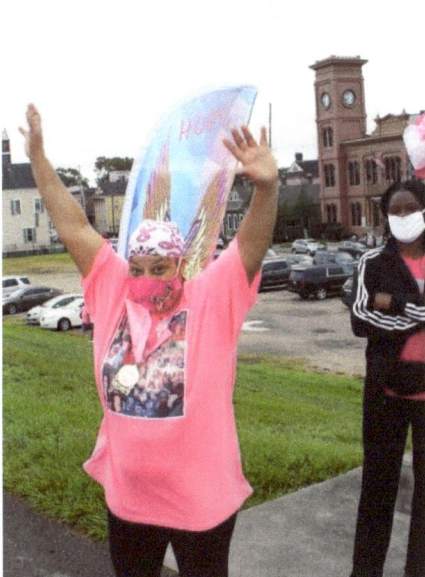

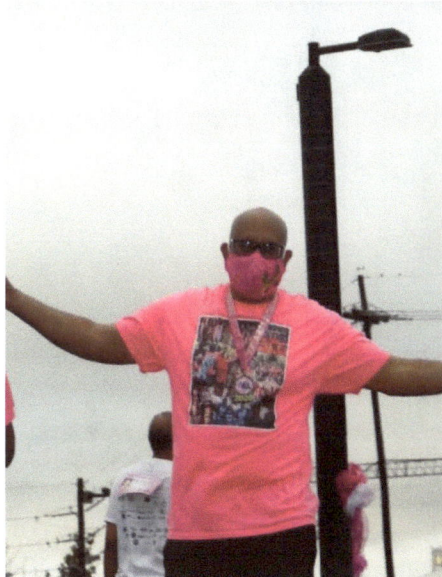

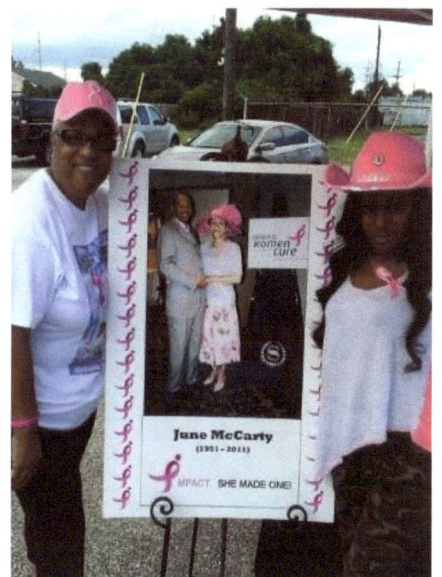

June McCarty

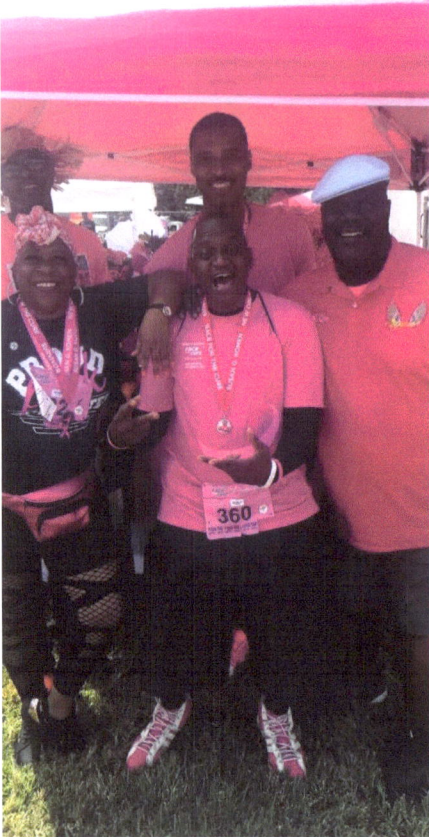

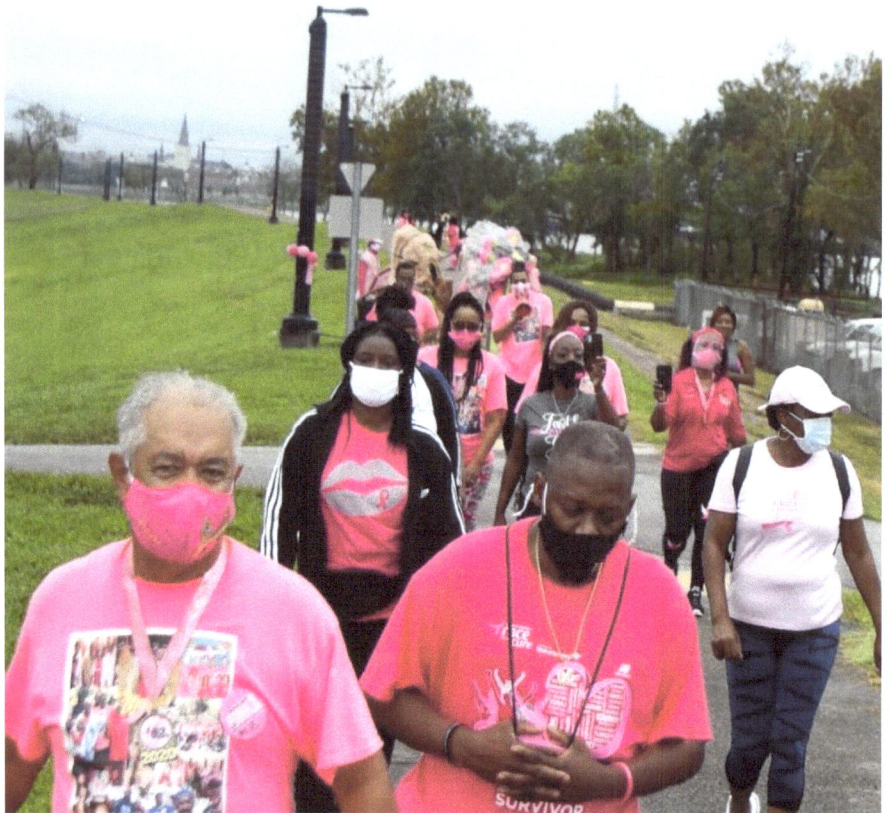

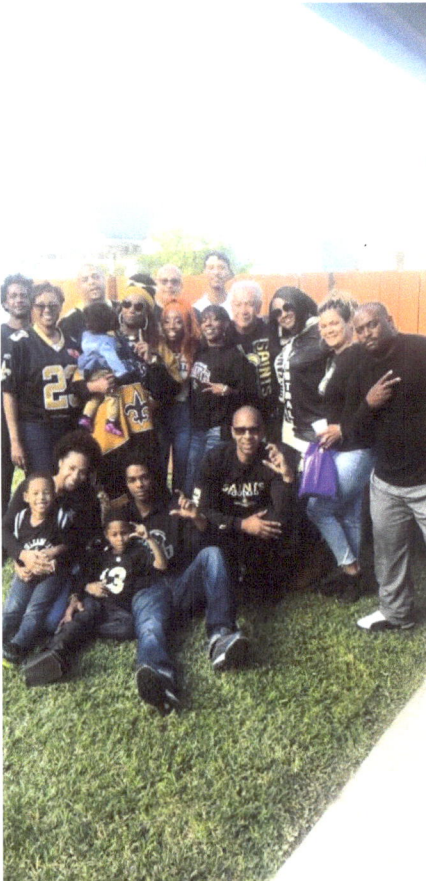

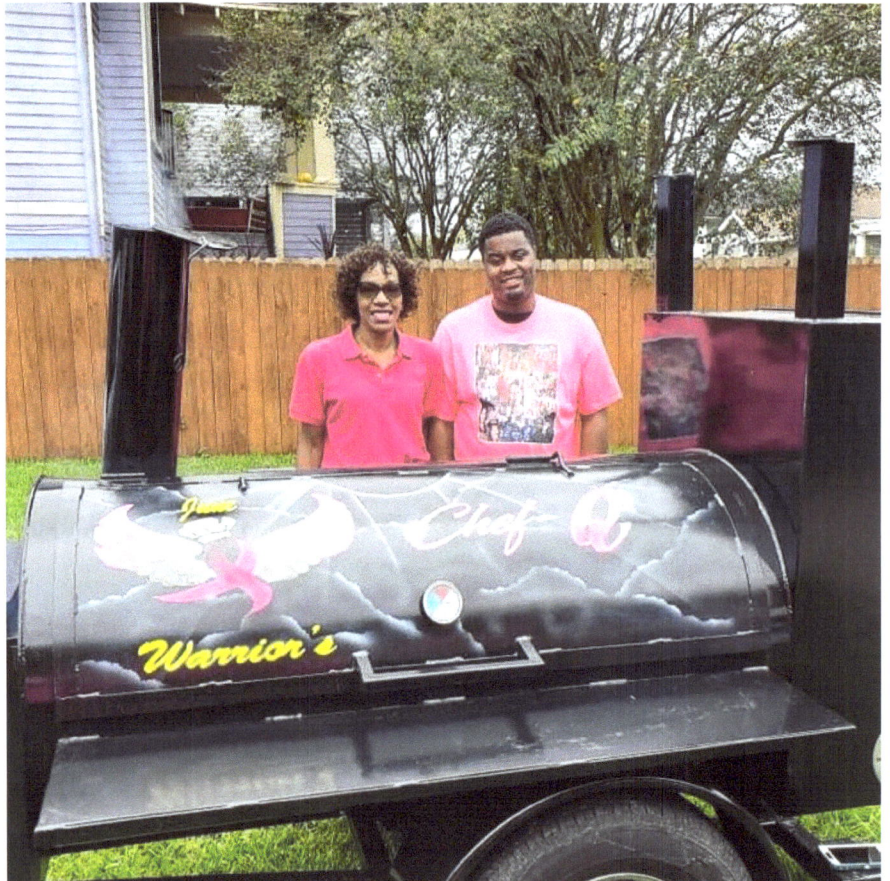

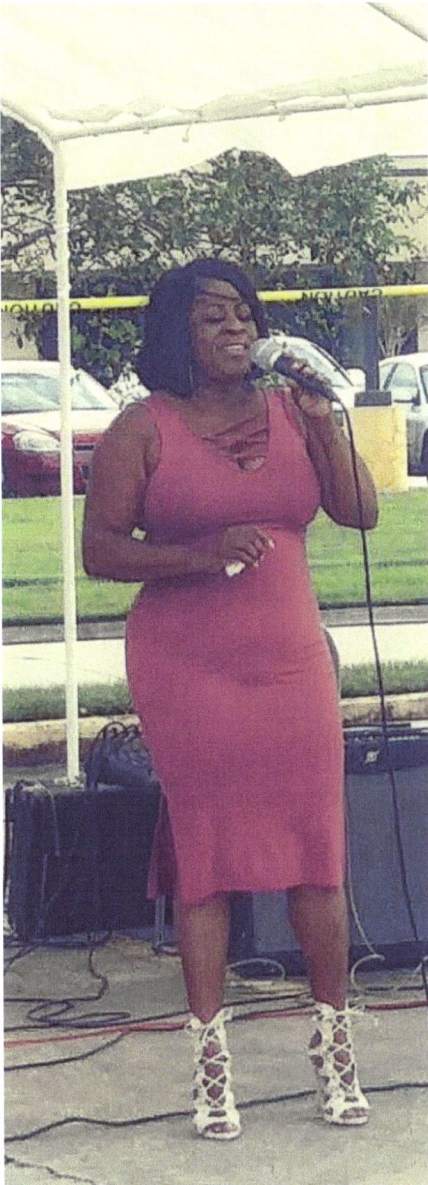

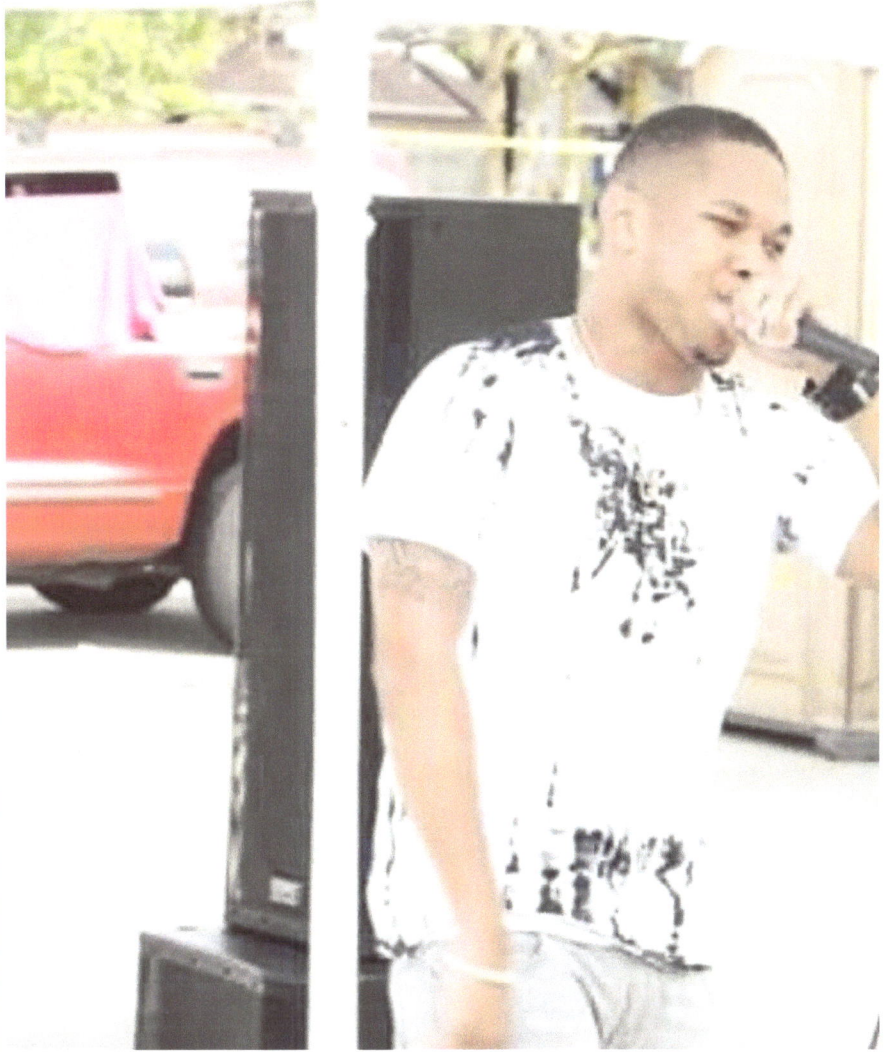

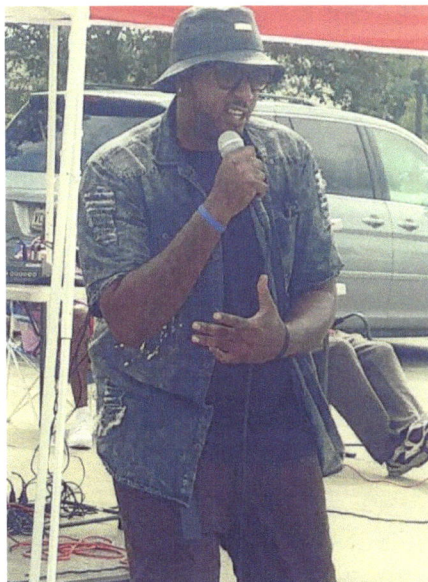

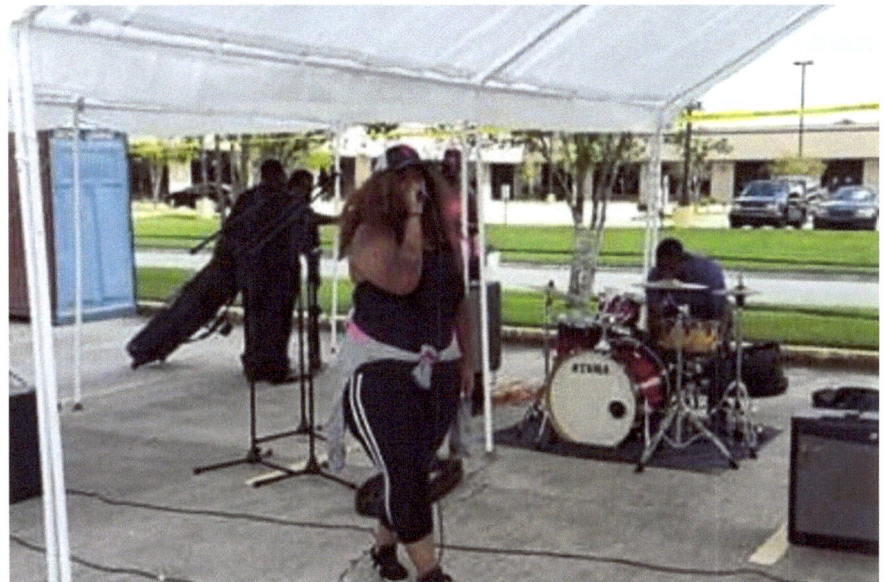

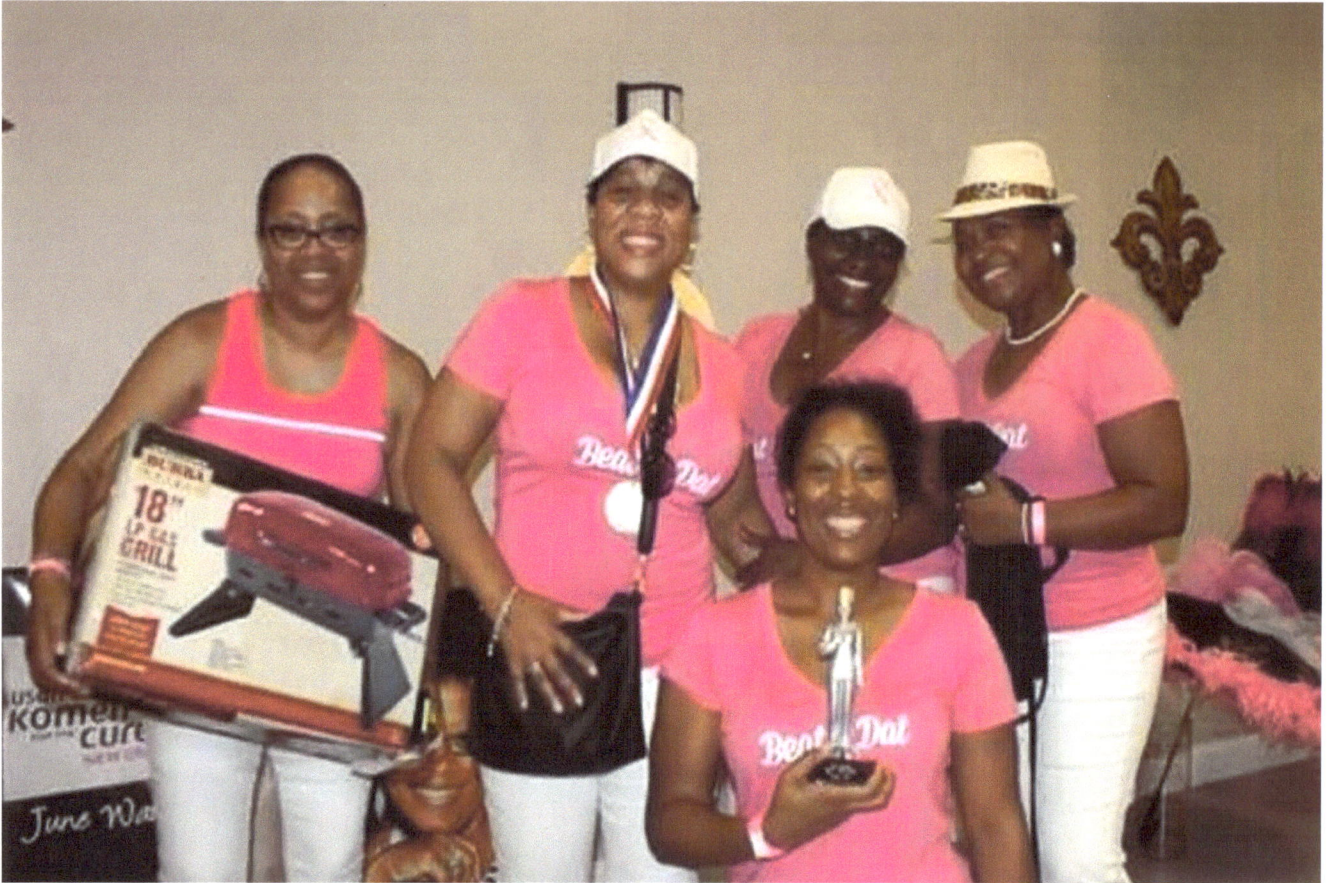

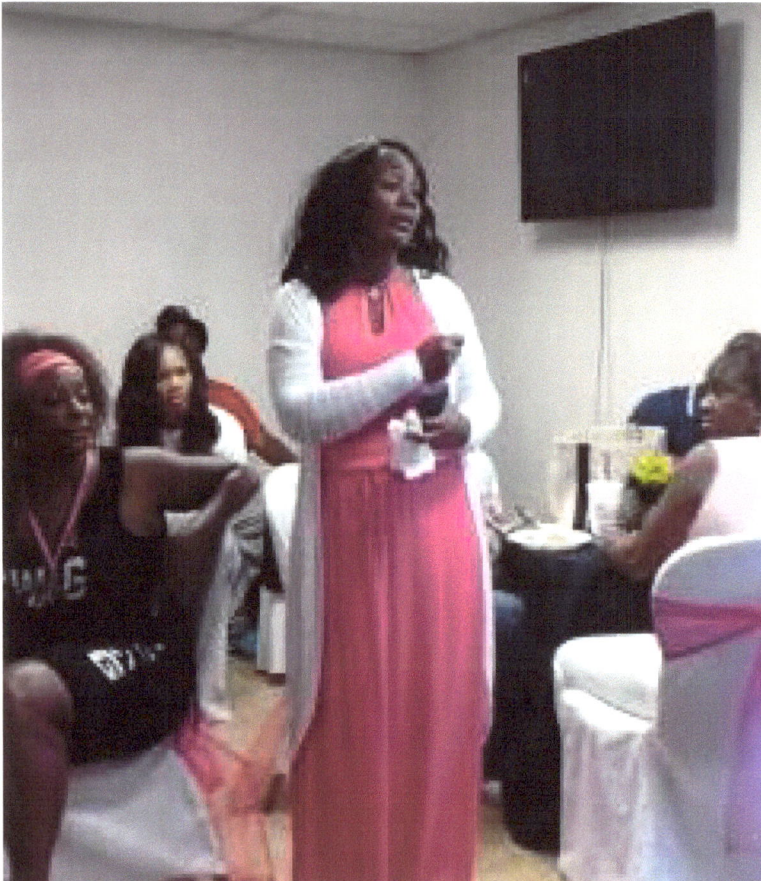

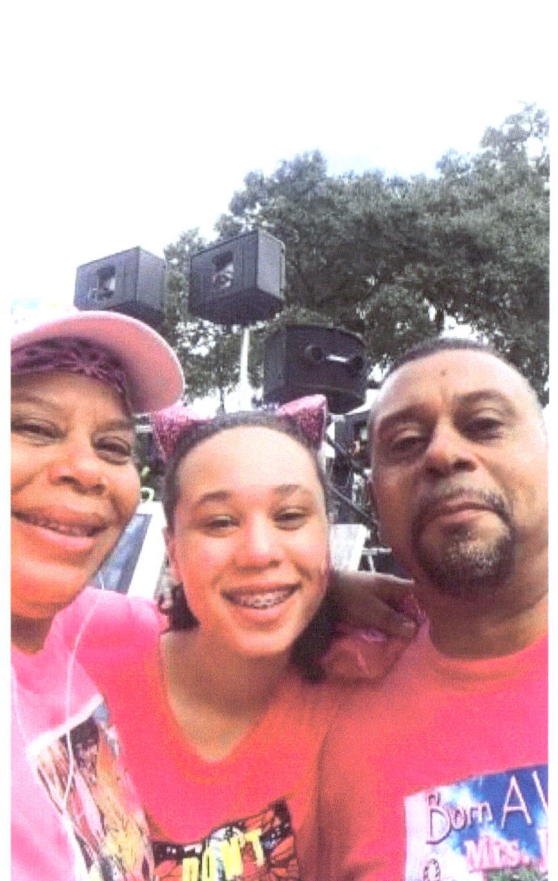

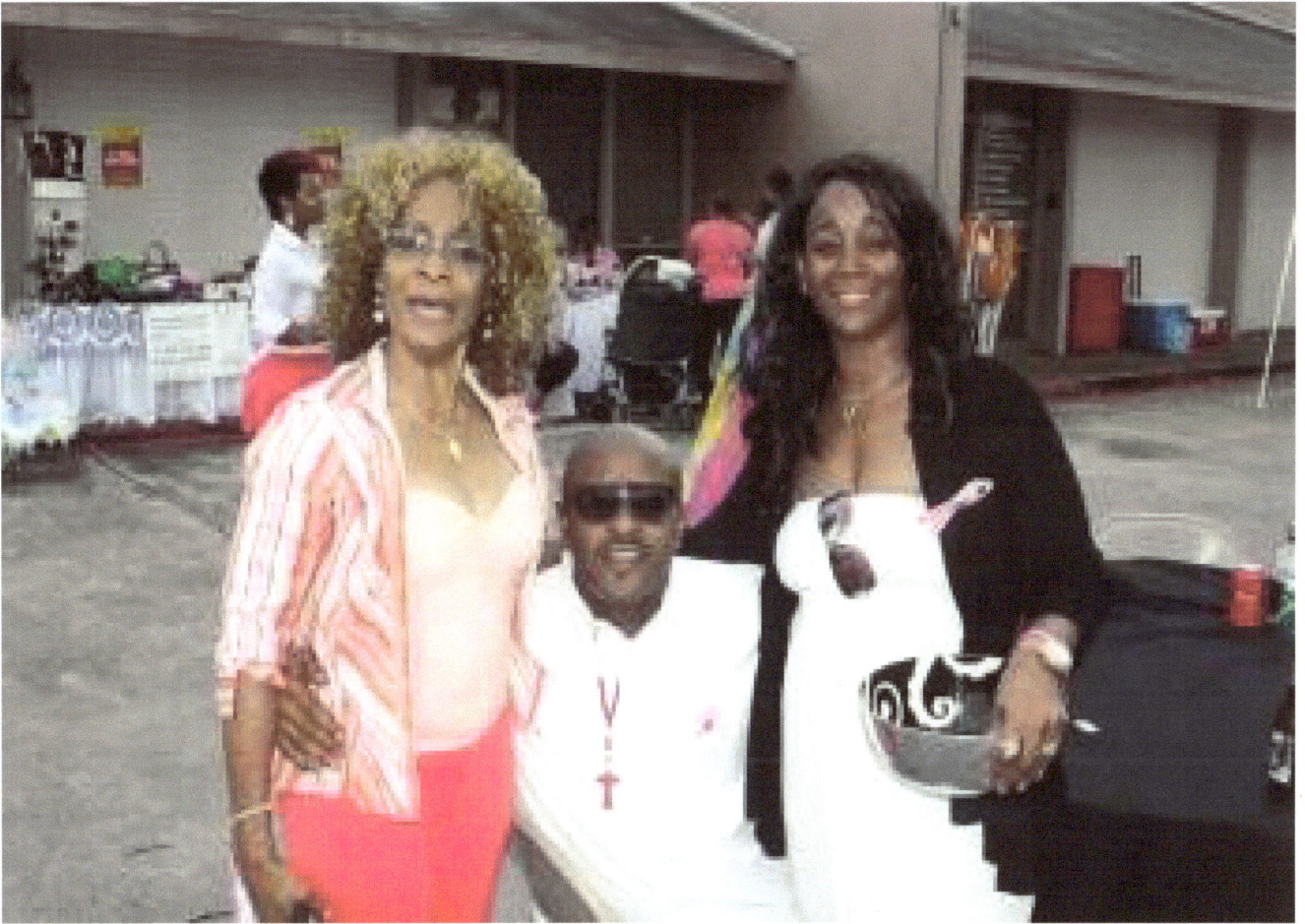

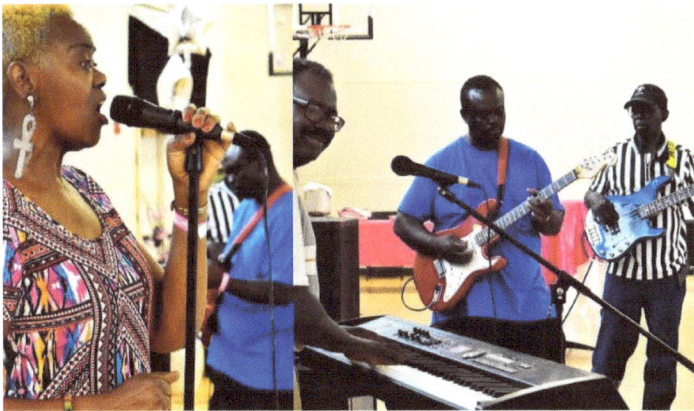

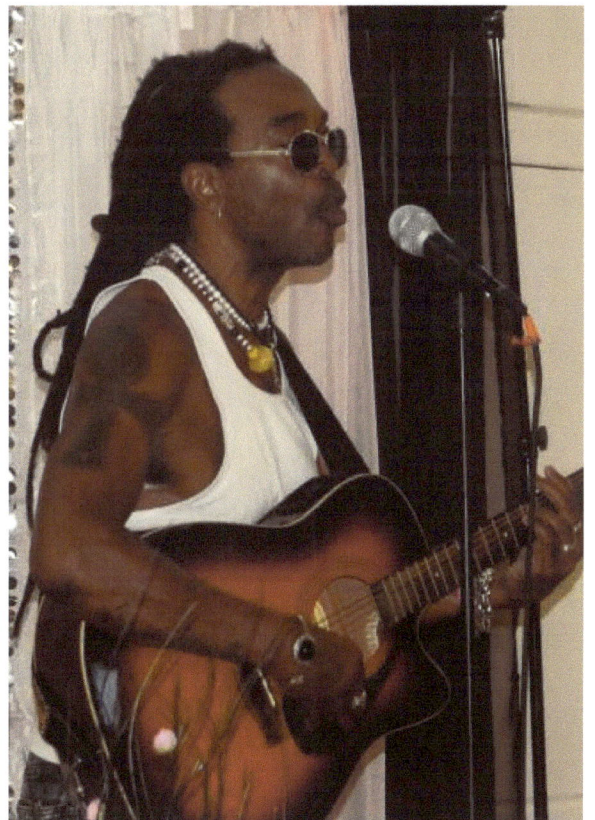

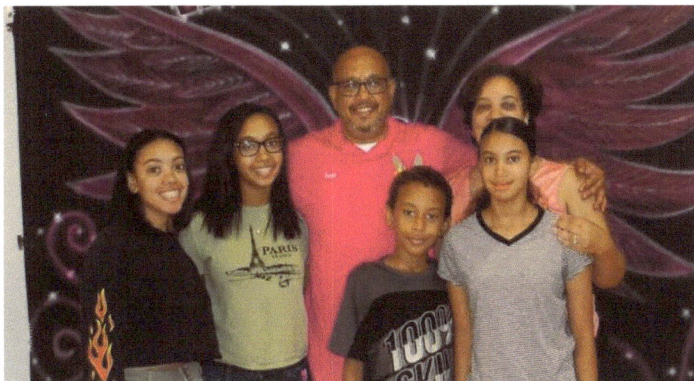

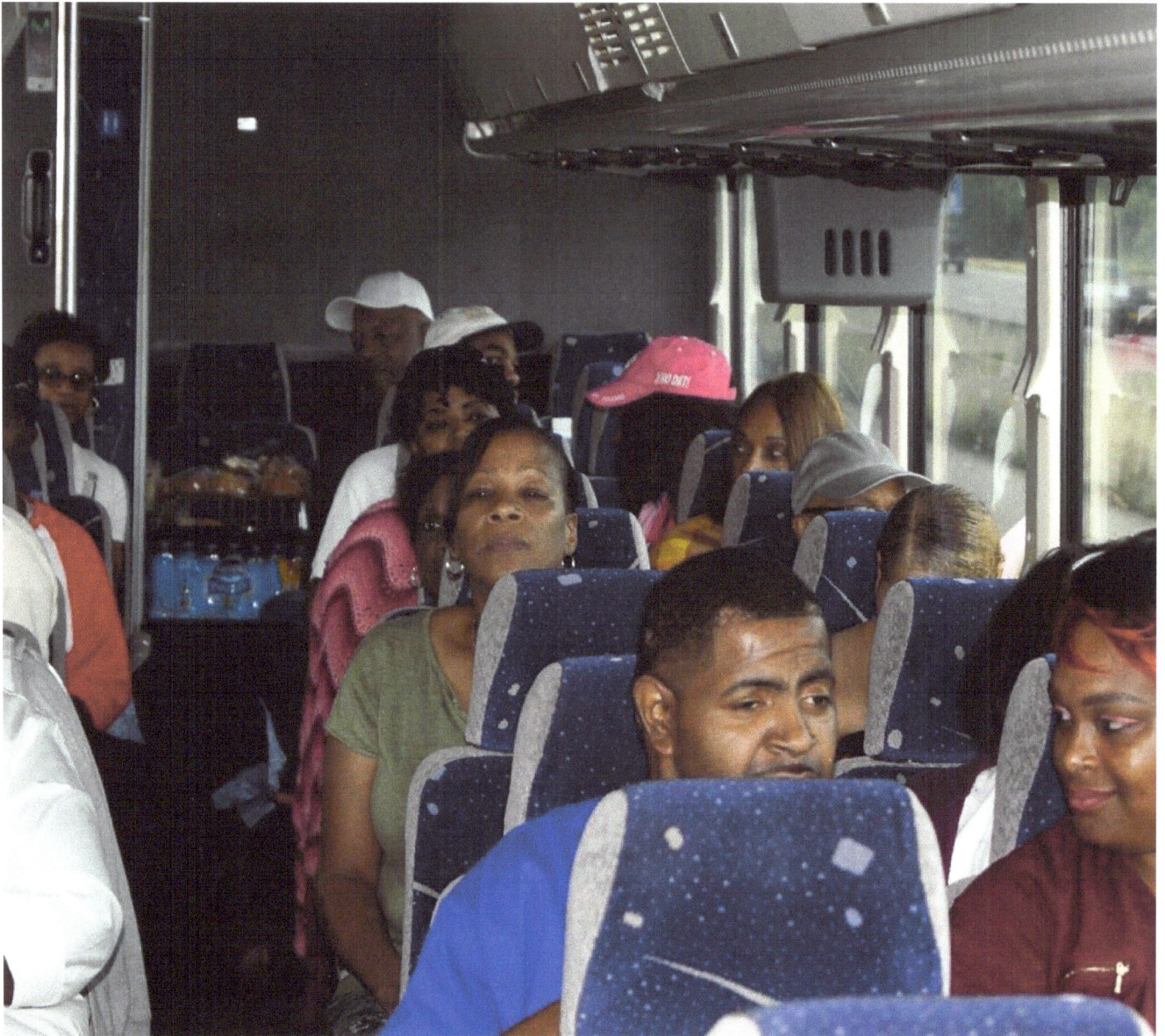

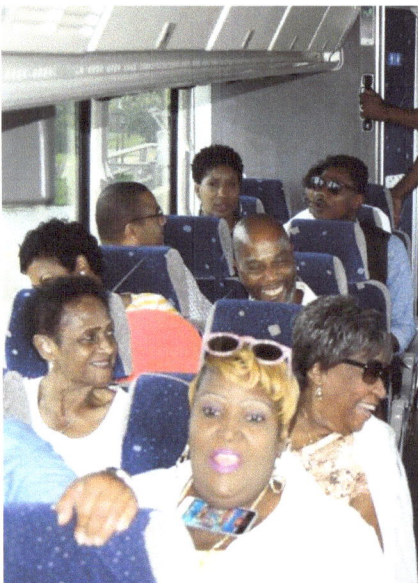

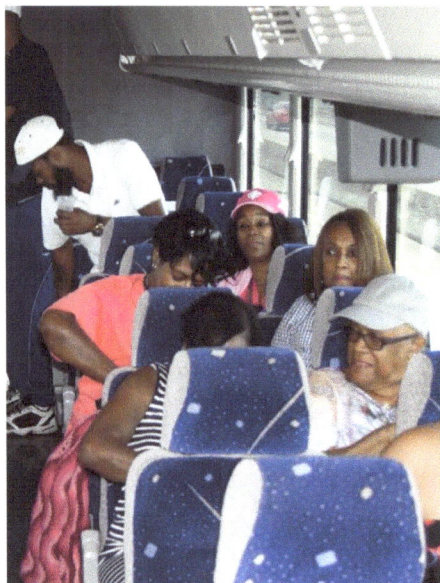

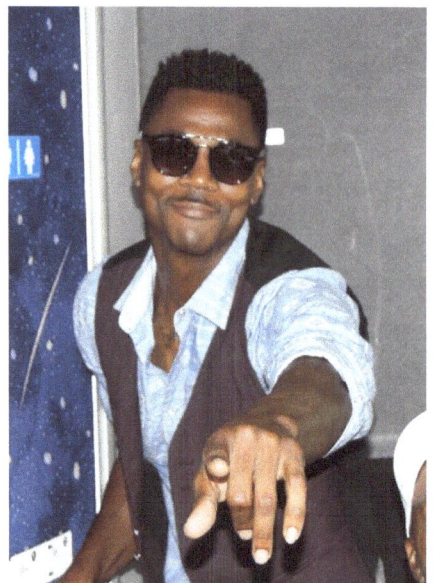

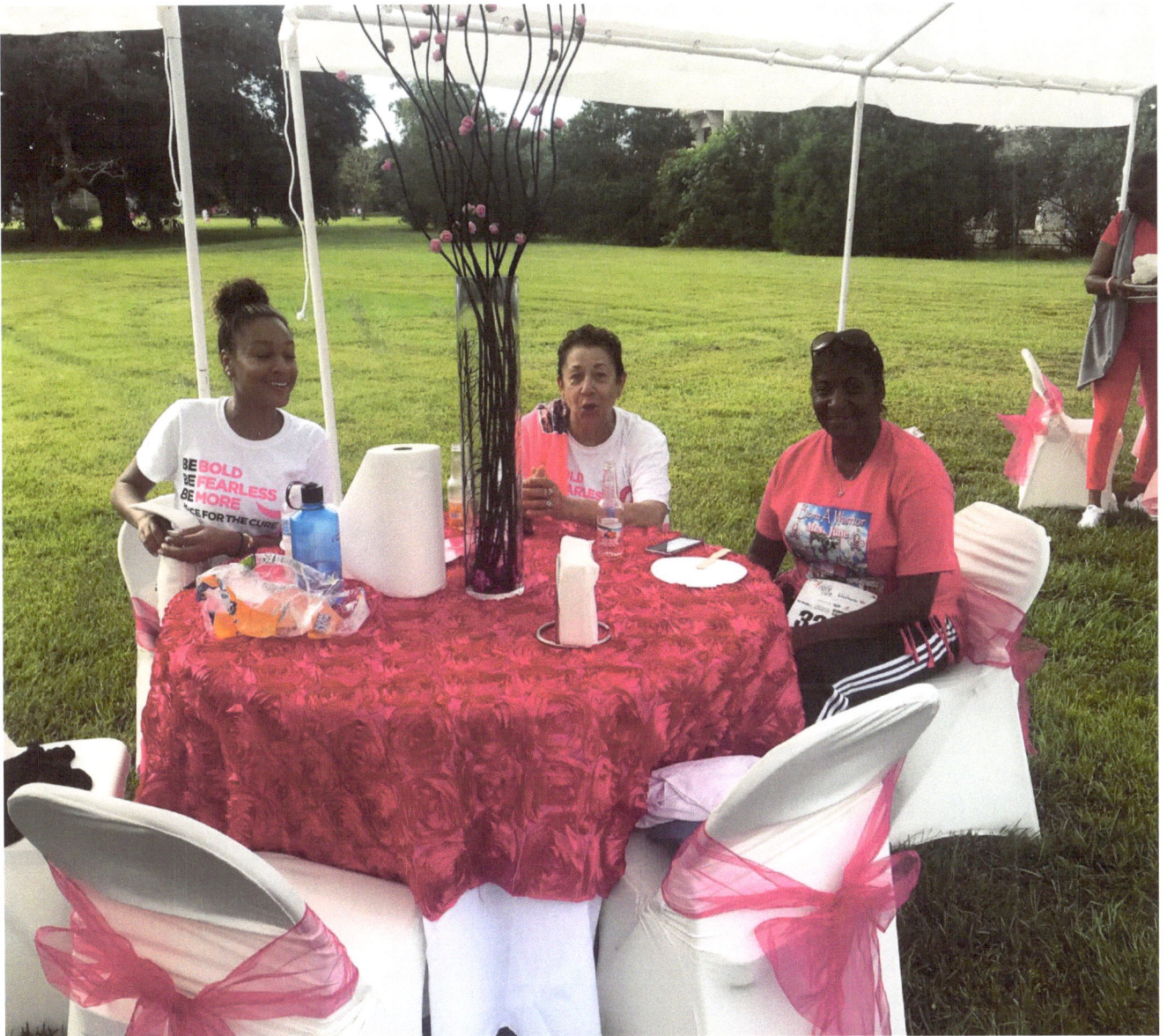

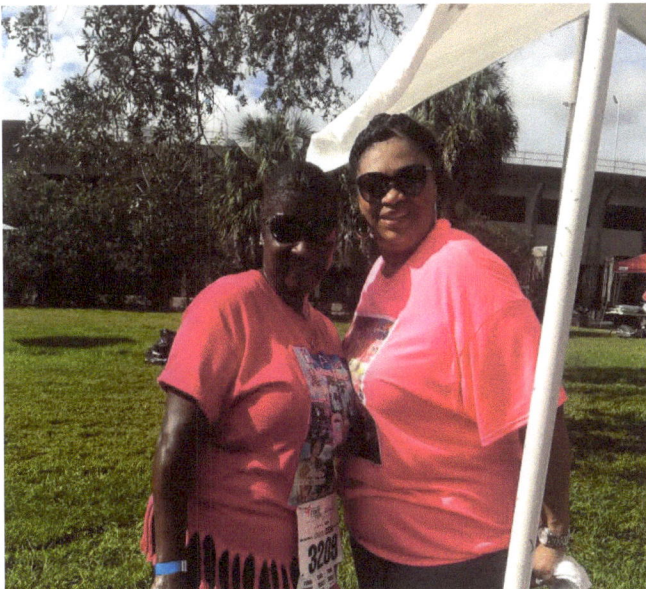

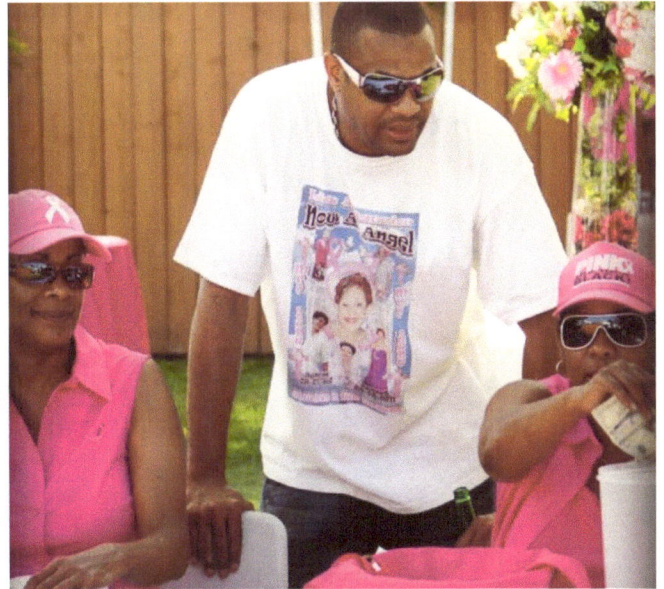

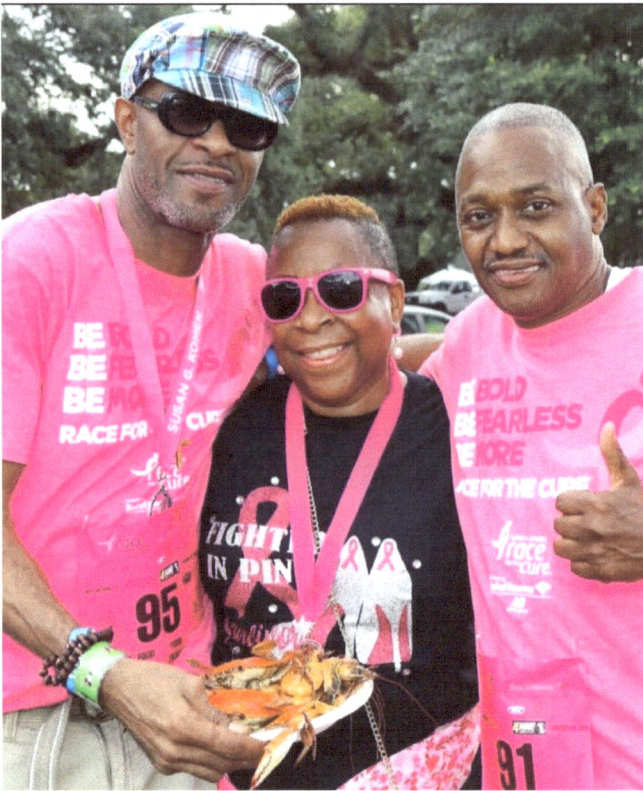

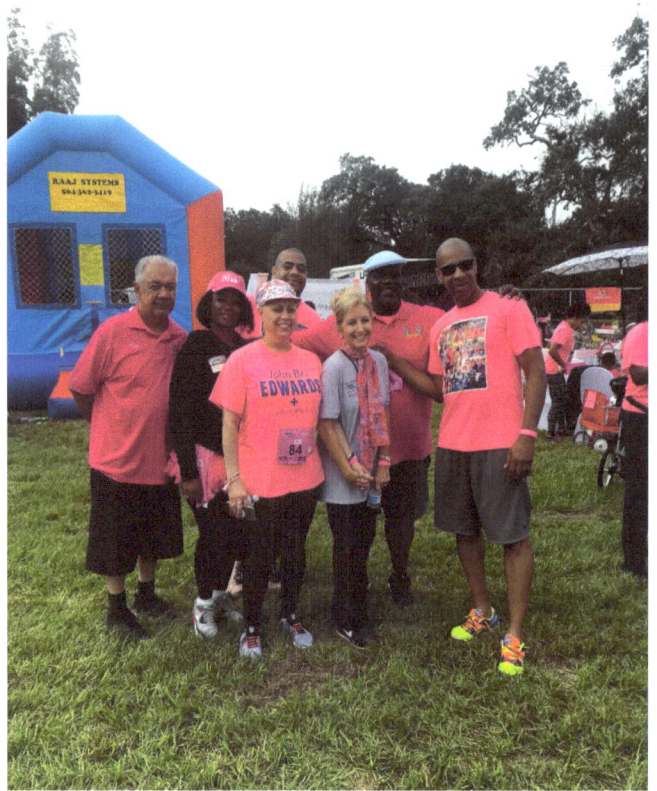

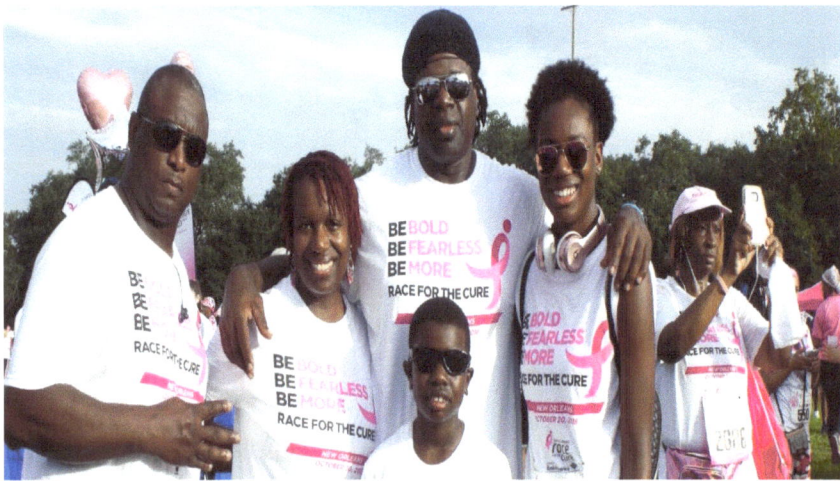

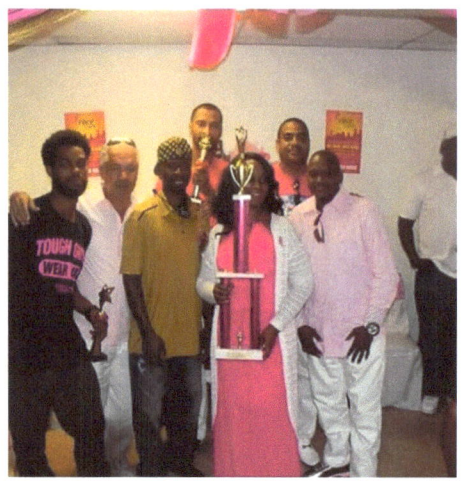

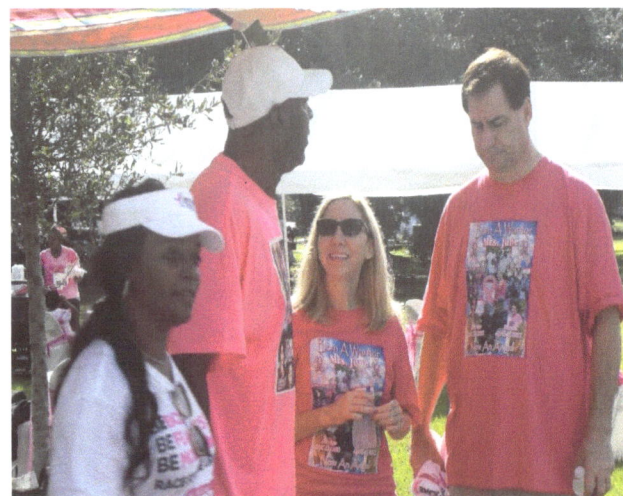

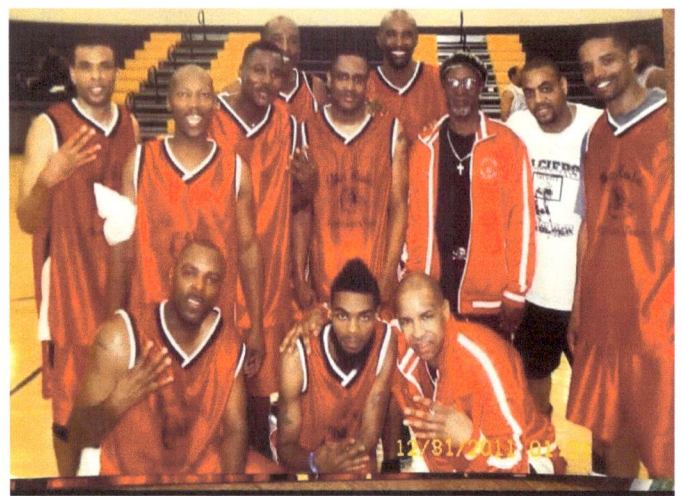

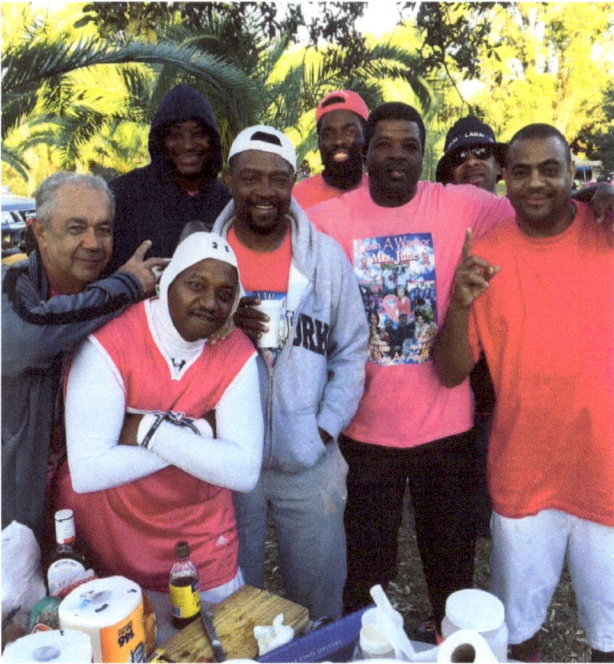

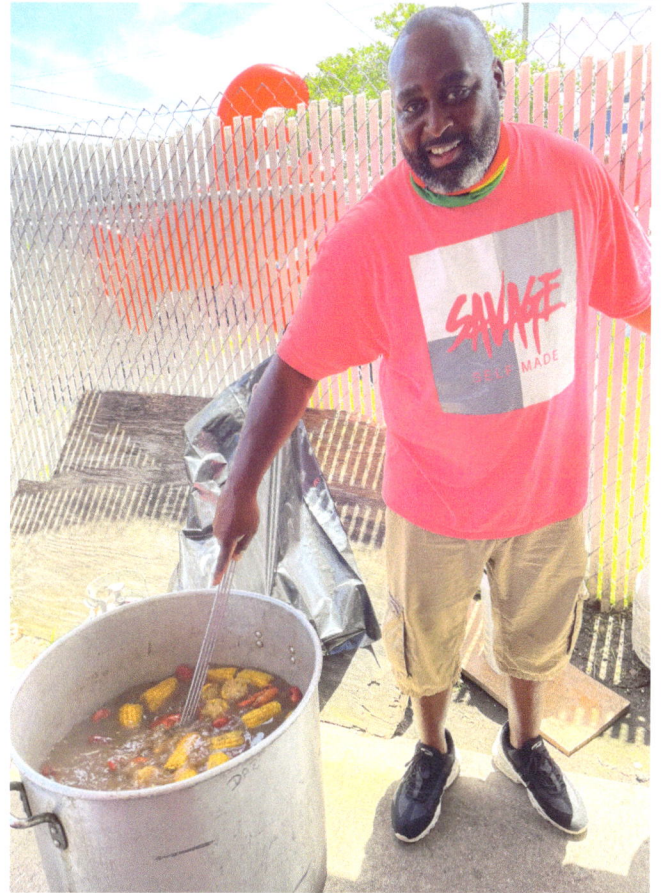

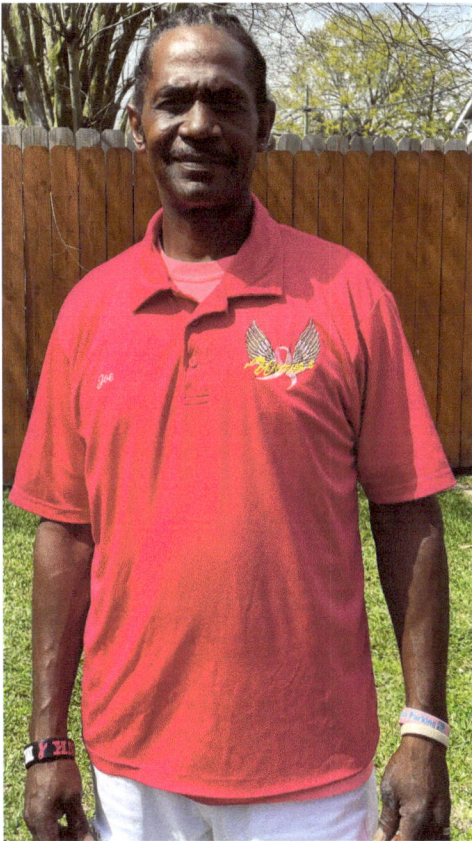

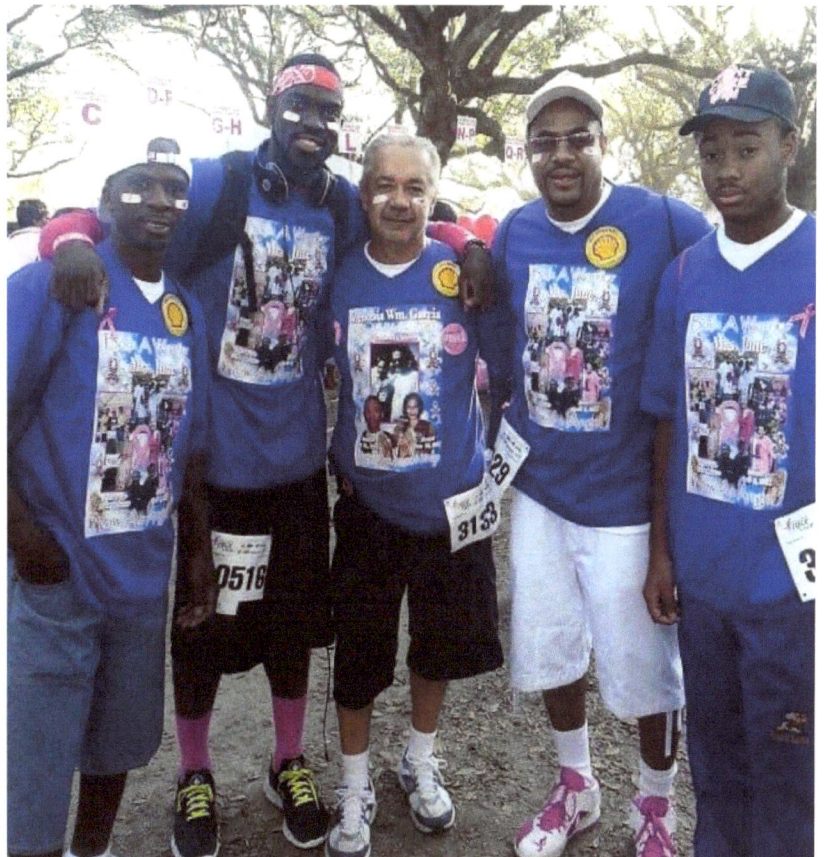

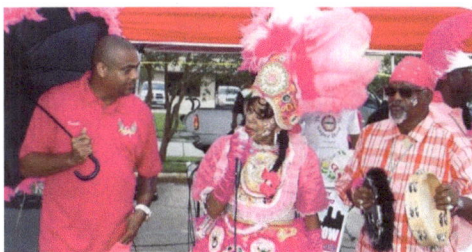

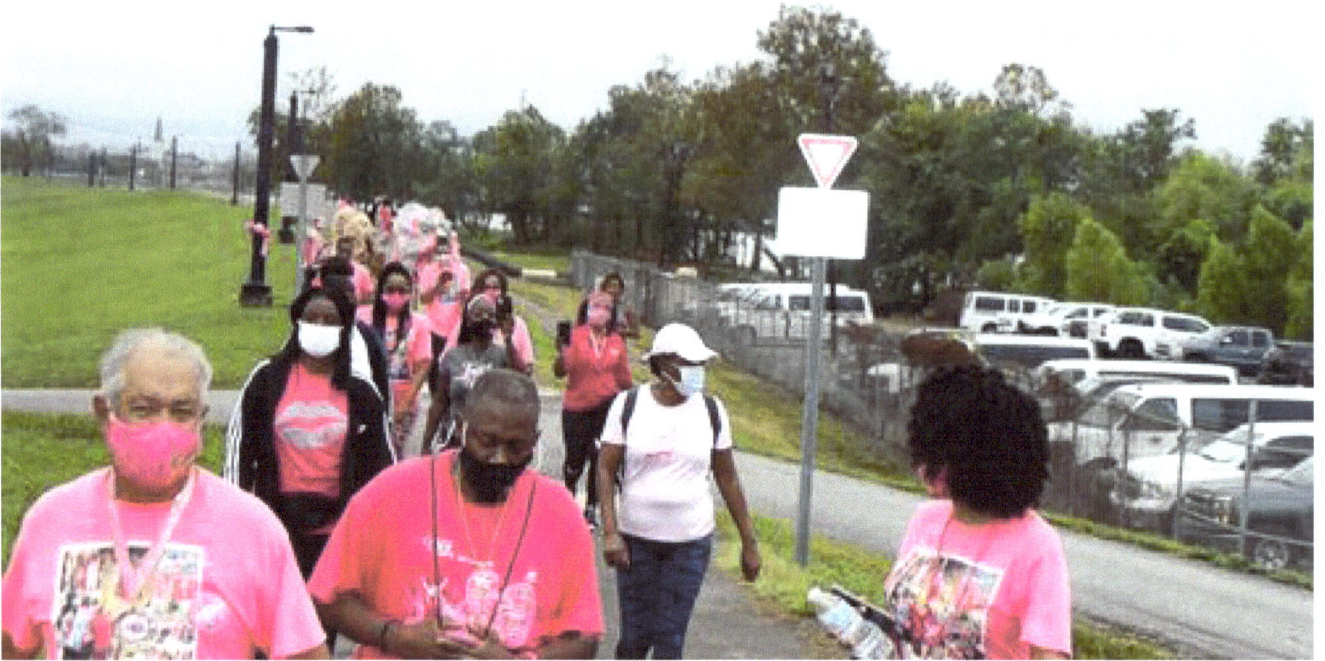

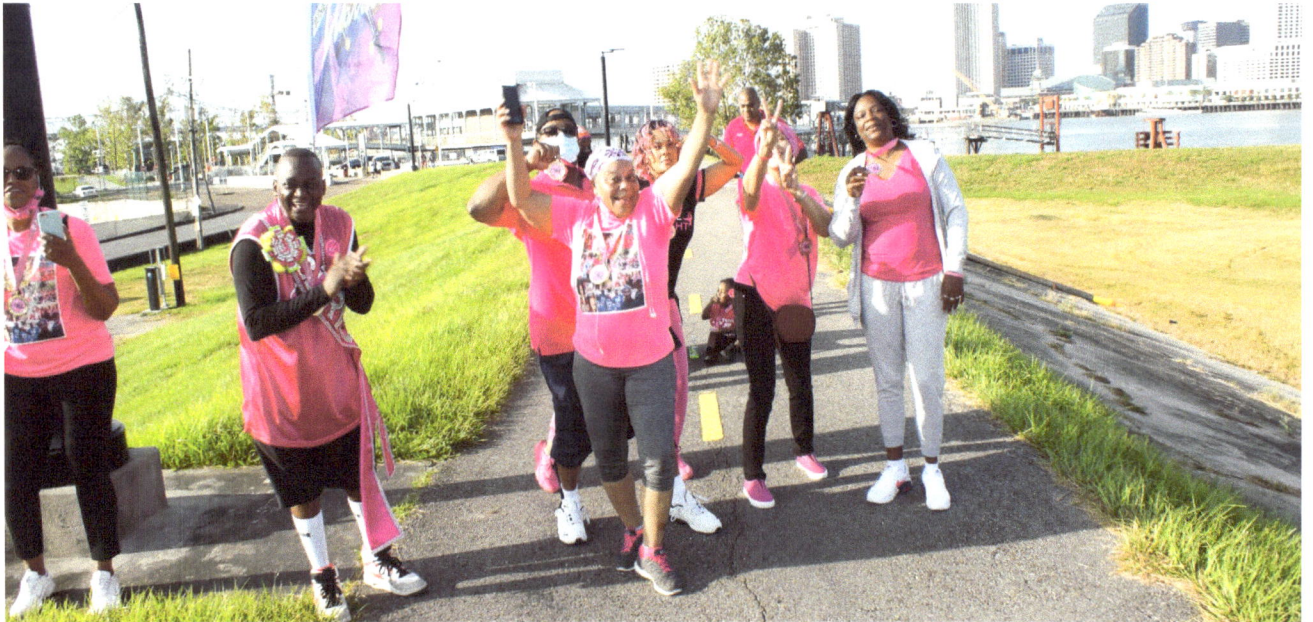

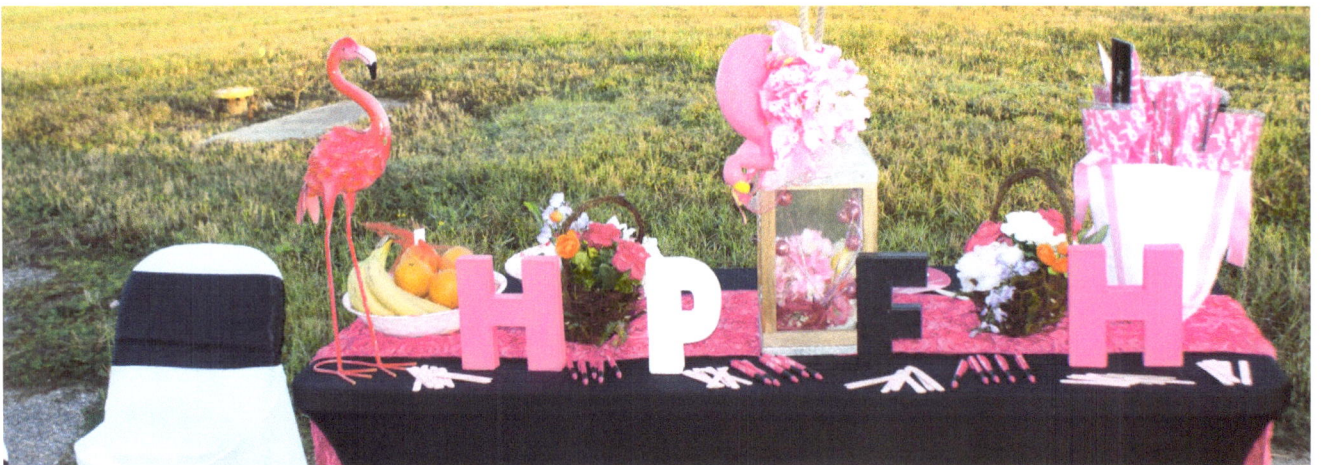

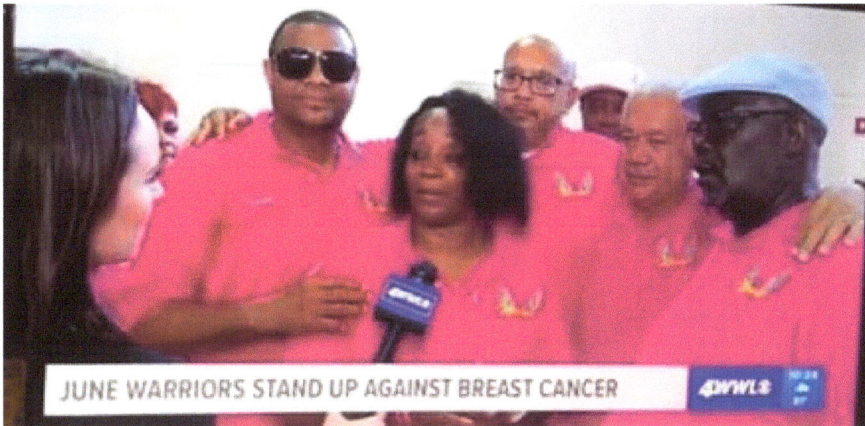

JUNE WARRIORS STAND UP AGAINST BREAST CANCER

We were covered by 4WWL news media for the Gumbo contest 2019, and the work we do.

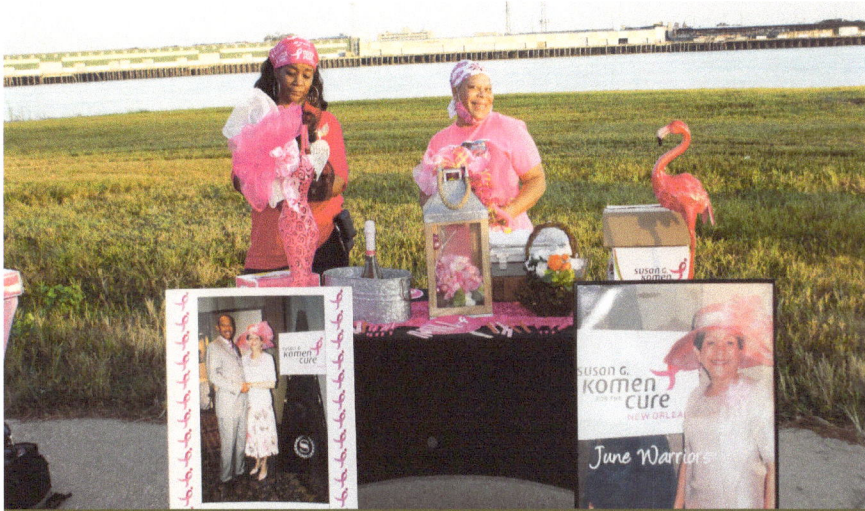

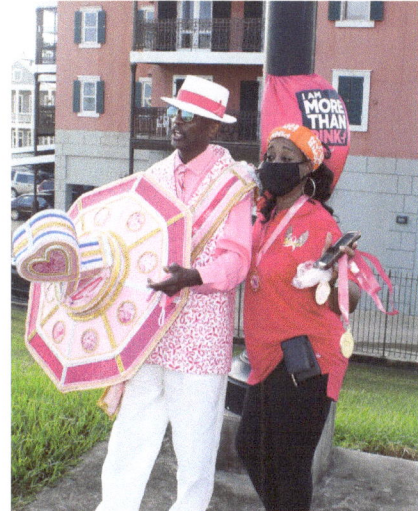

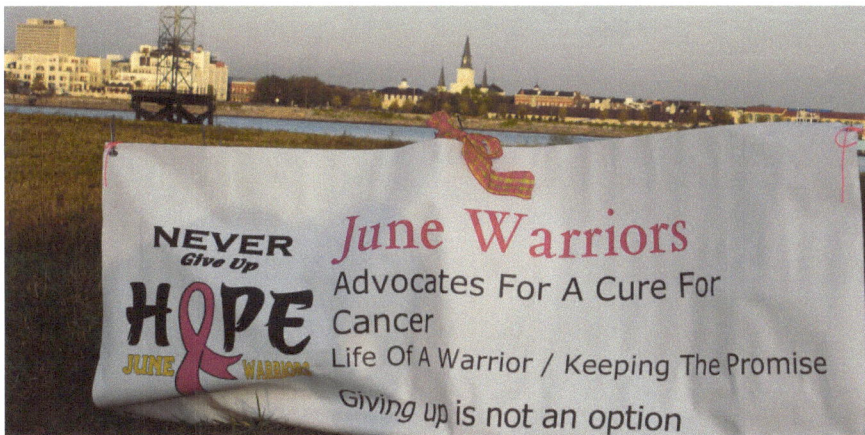

NEVER Give Up
H❤PE
JUNE WARRIORS

June Warriors
Advocates For A Cure For Cancer
Life Of A Warrior / Keeping The Promise

Giving up is not an option

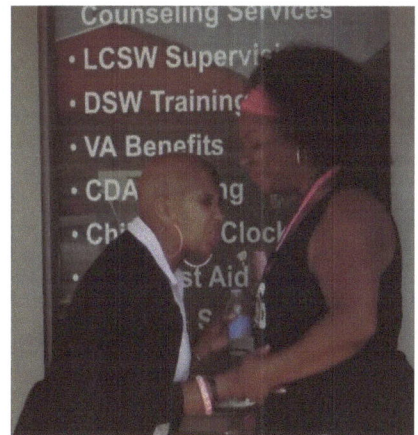

Counseling Services
• LCSW Supervis
• DSW Training
• VA Benefits
• CDA
• Chi   Clock

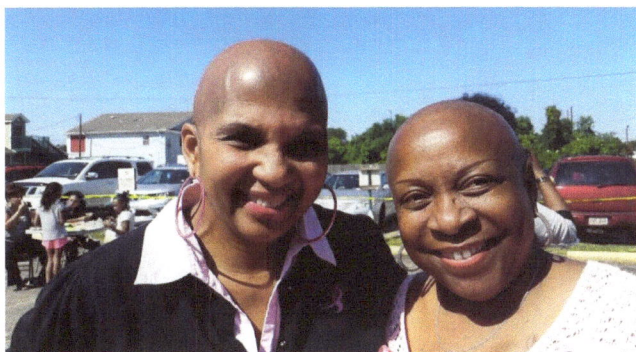

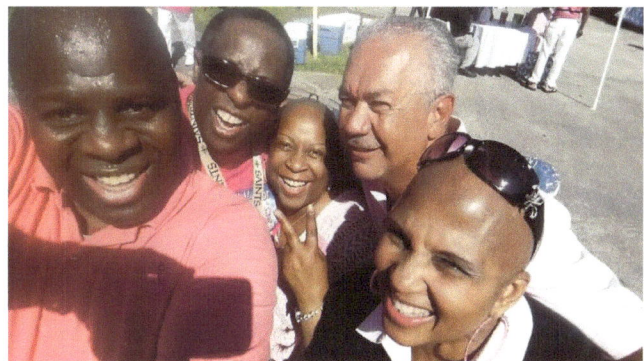

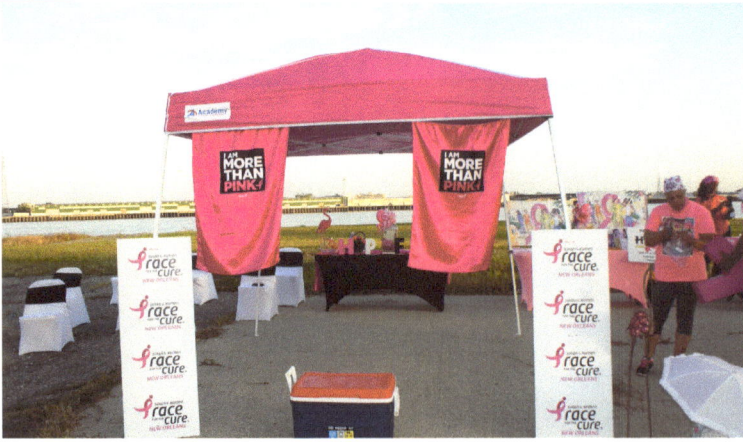
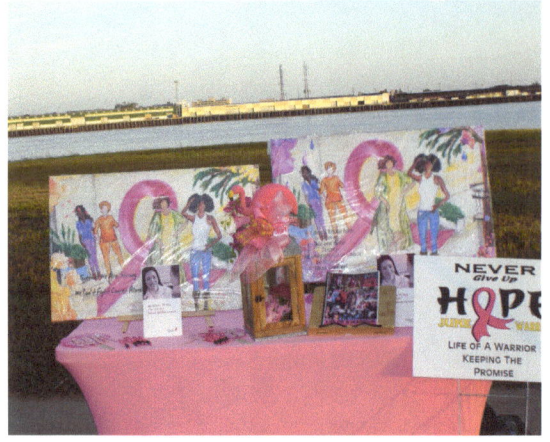
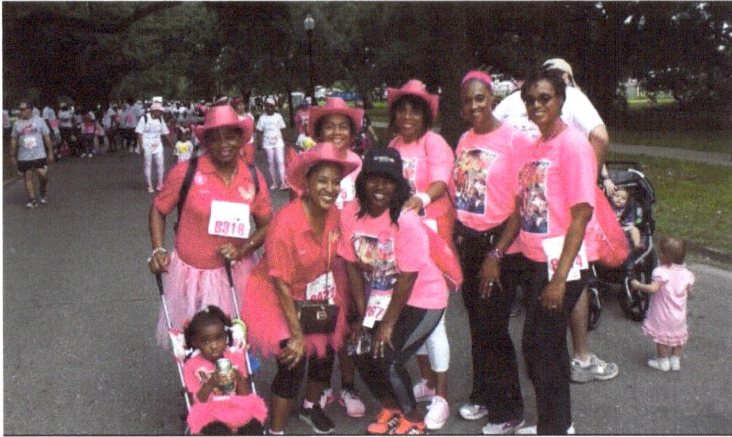
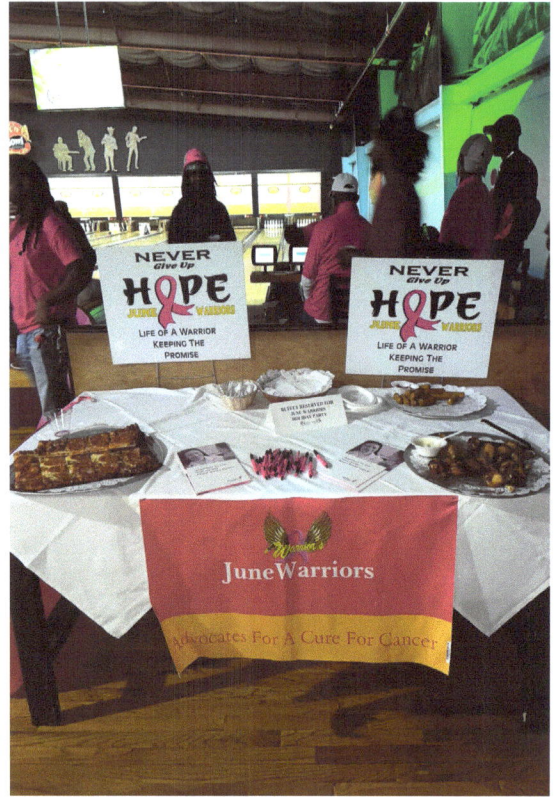
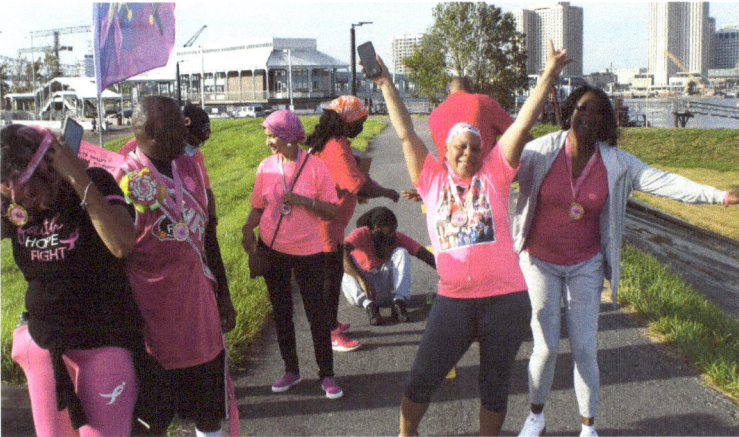
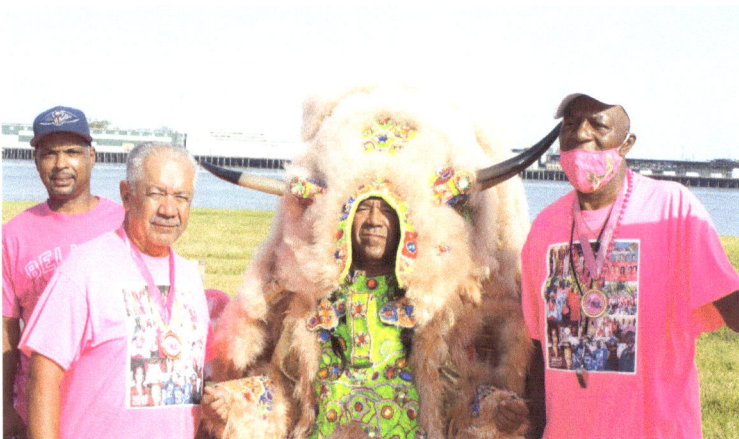
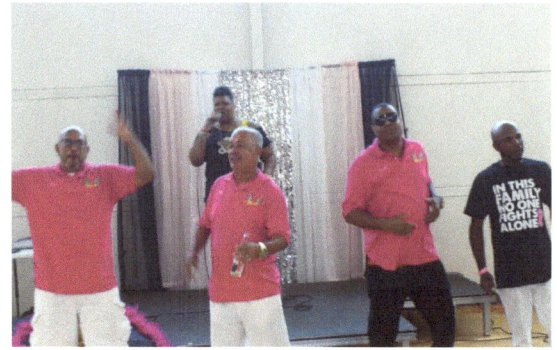

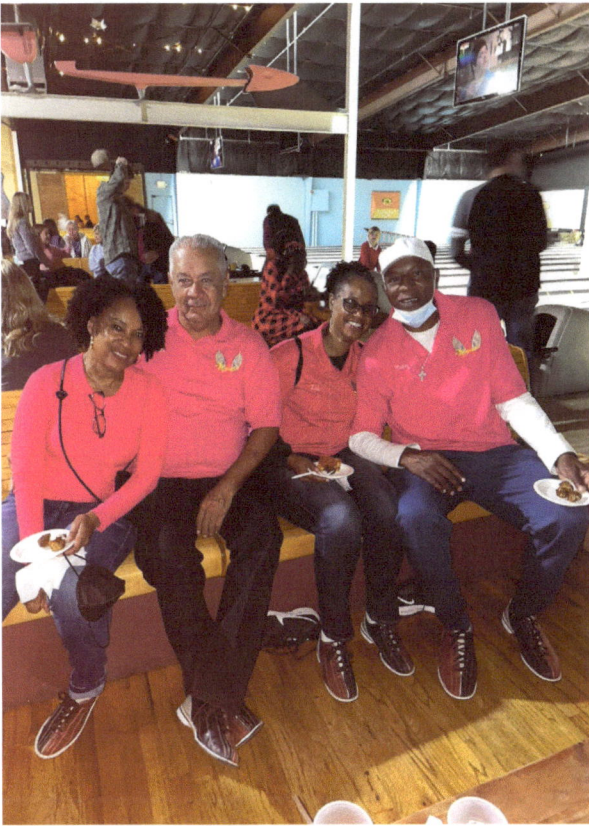

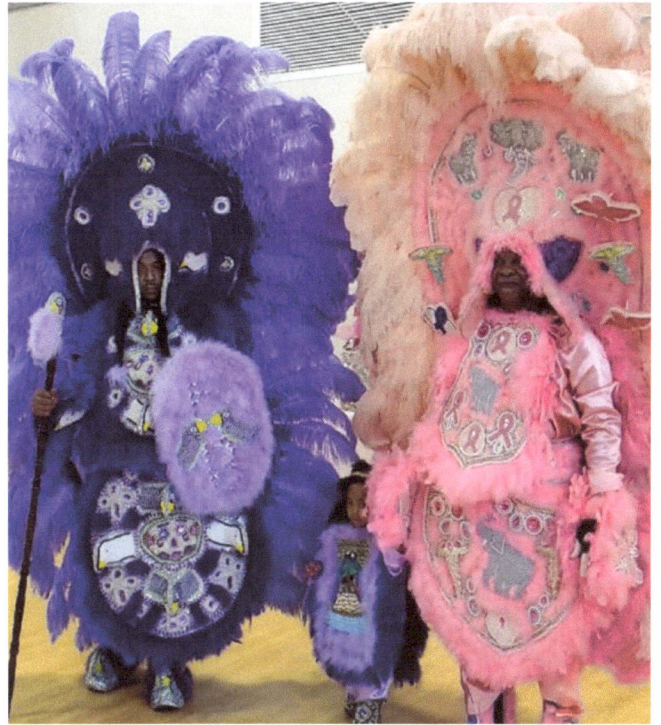

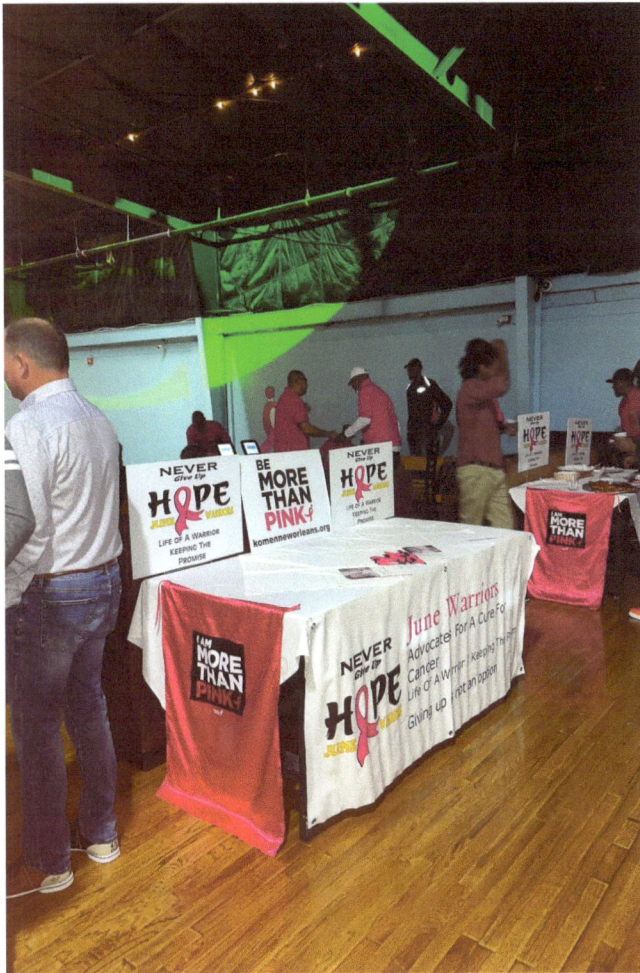

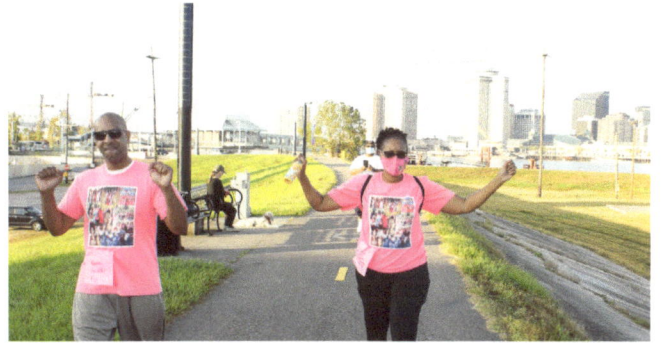

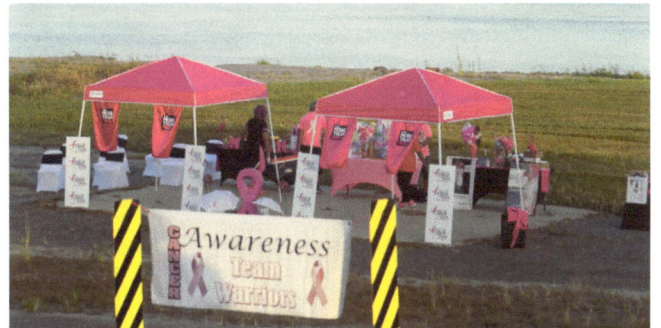

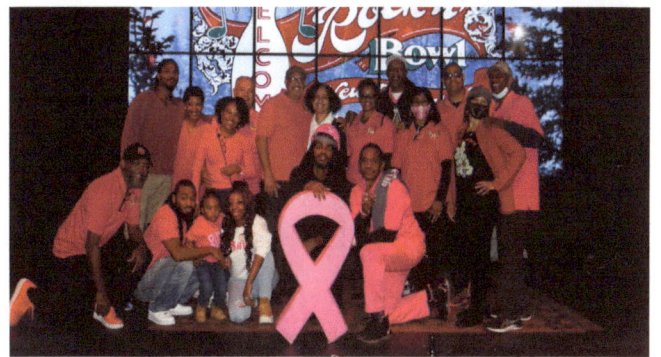

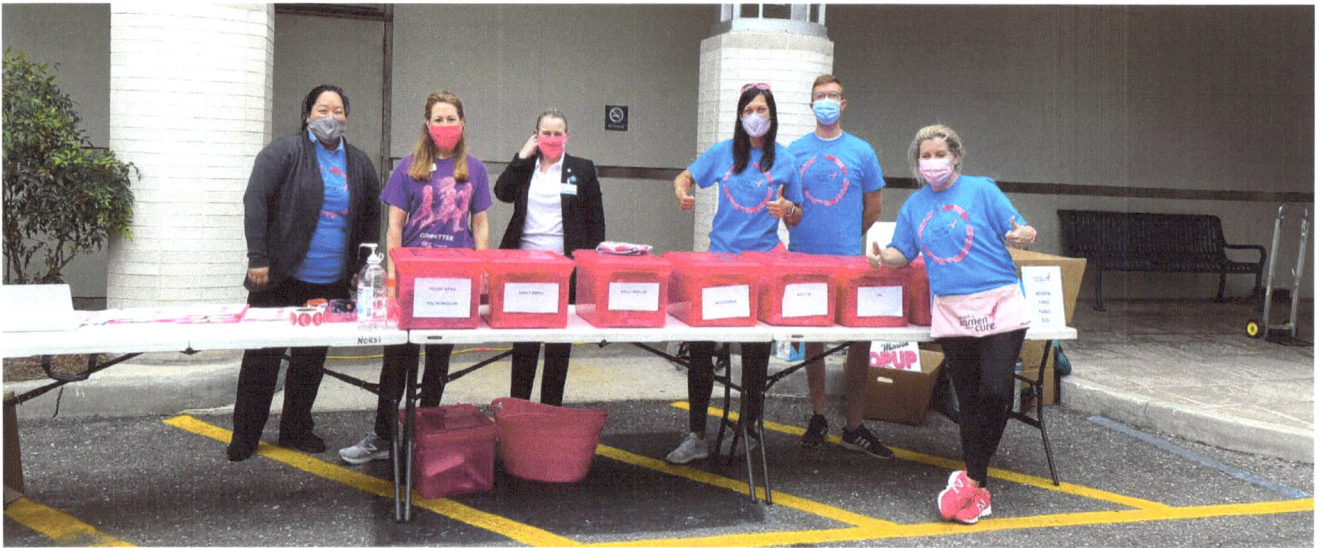

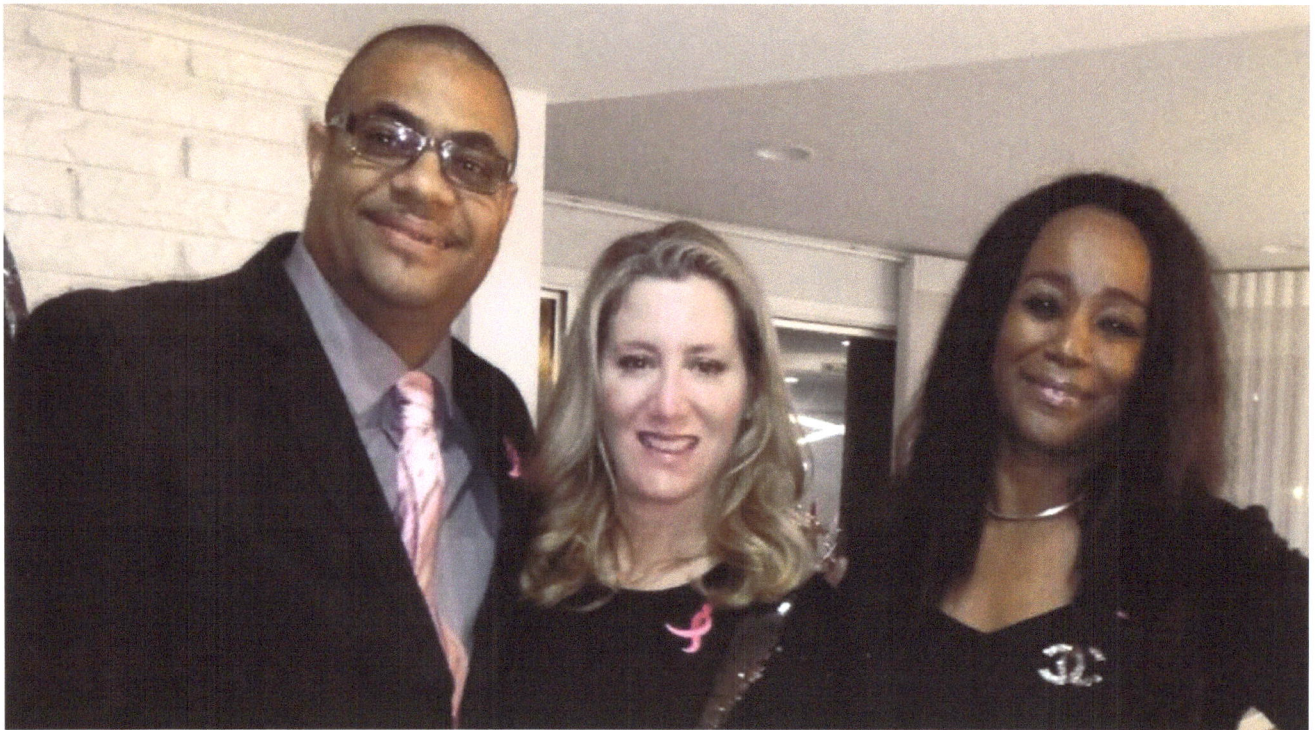

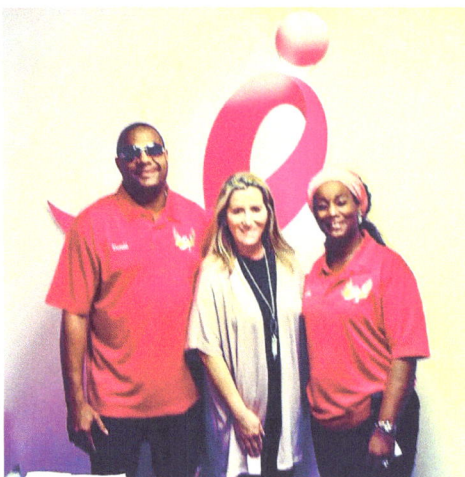

June Warrior's Donald and Demetris Price with Lisa Plunkett/Executive Director of Susan G. Komen.

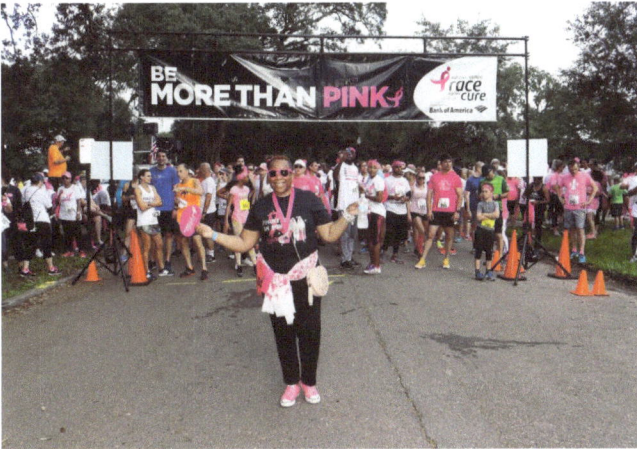

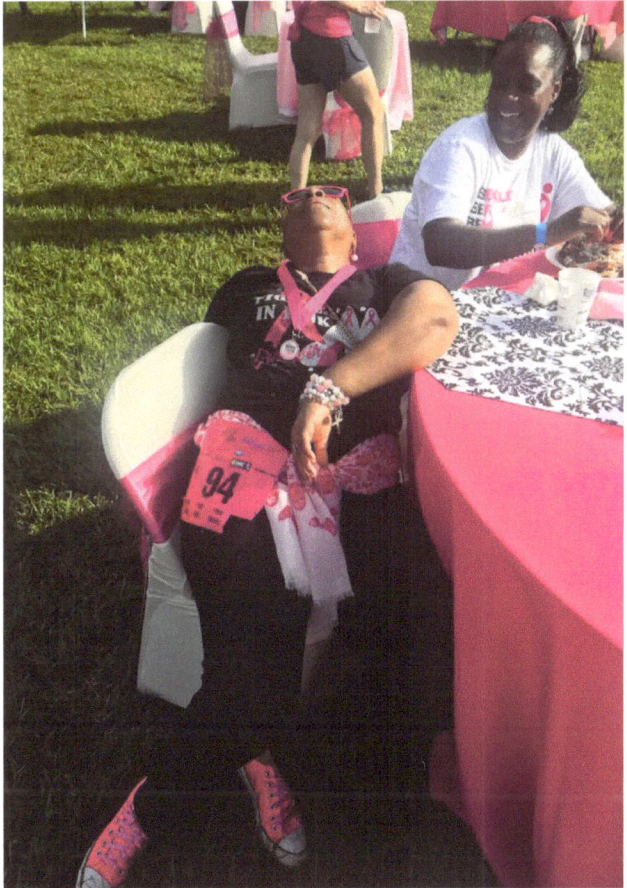

Joycelyn Duplessis was honored, and Donald Price was the volunteer of the year at the Race for the Cure 2018.

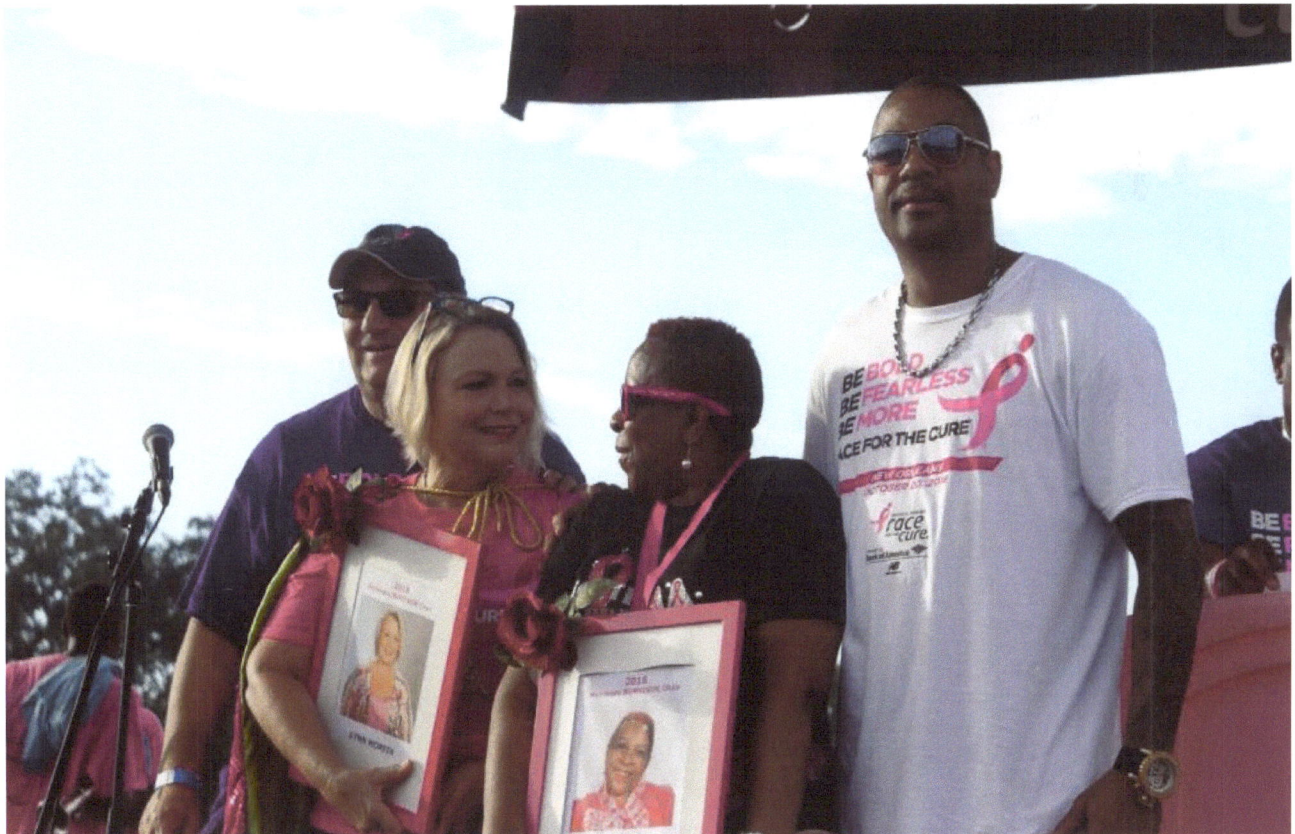

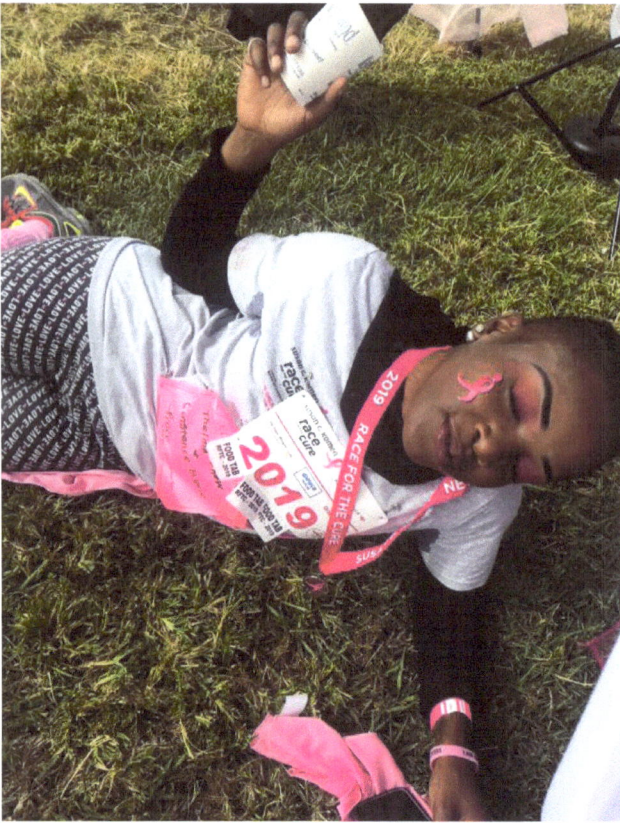

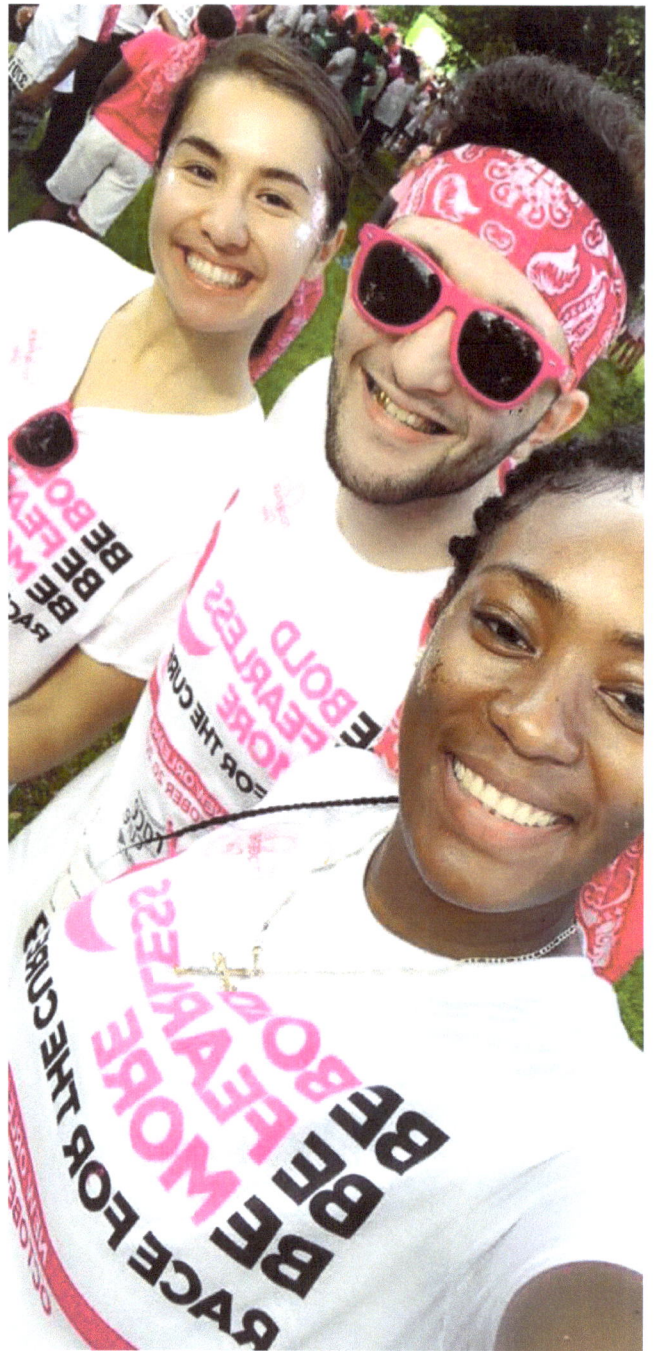

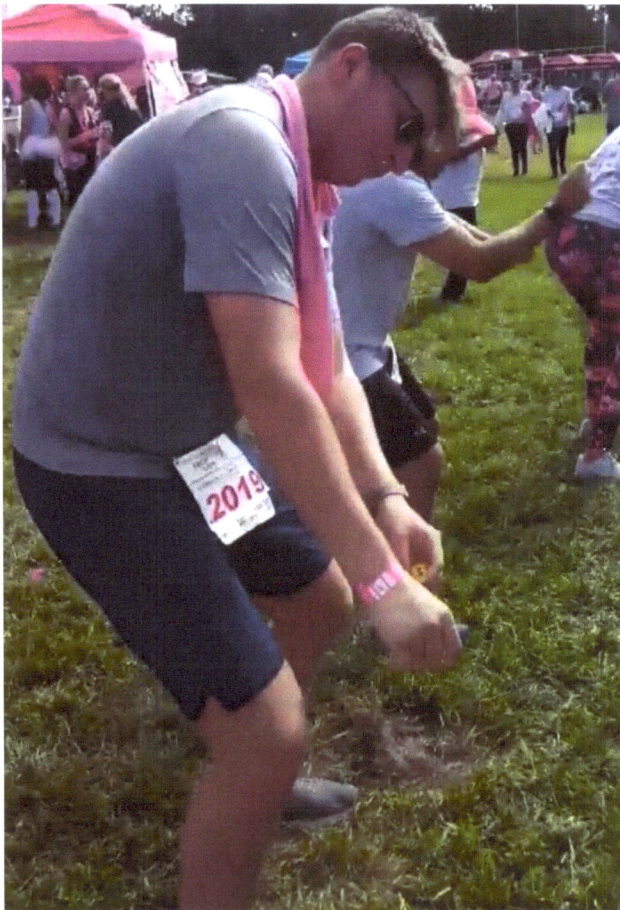

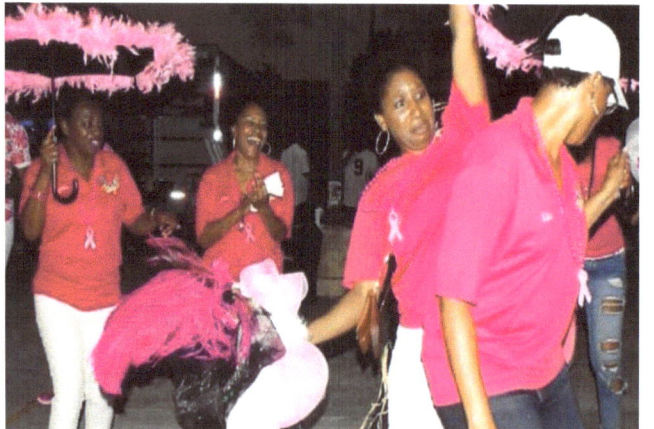

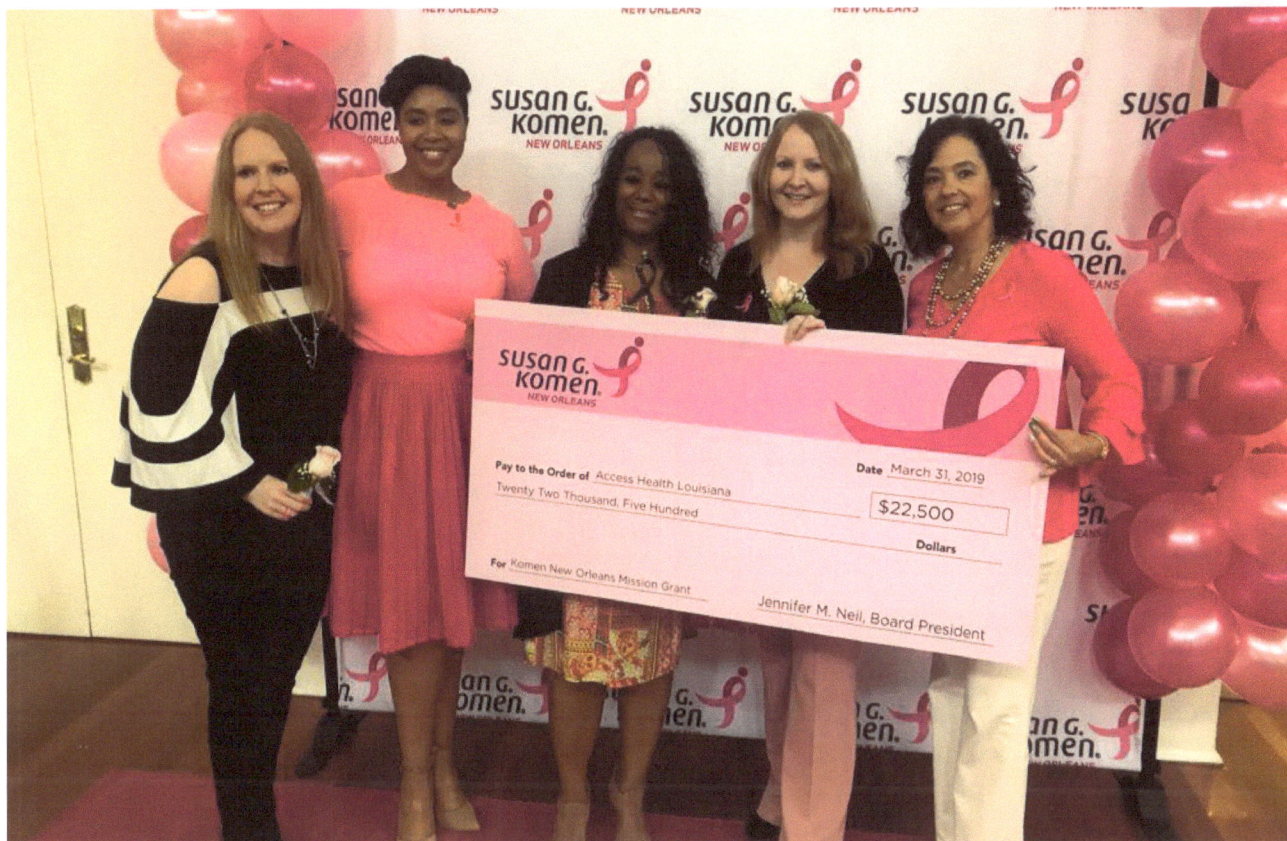

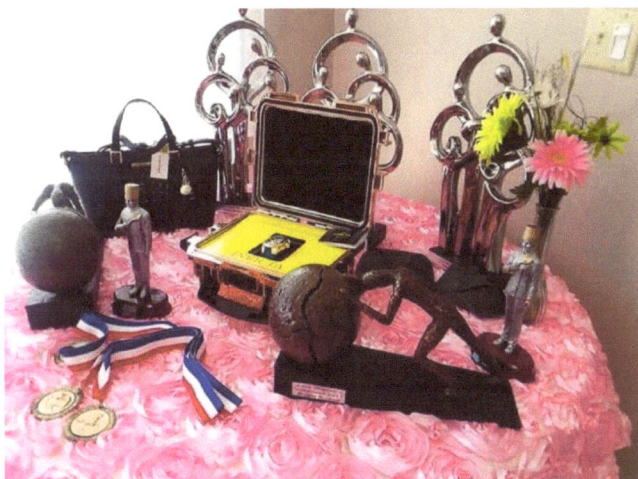

Top: *Demetris Price was honored at the volunteers' luncheon for Susan G. Komen 2019 and was able to participate in giving out the check to one of the participants of the grant that all the race group fundraise.*

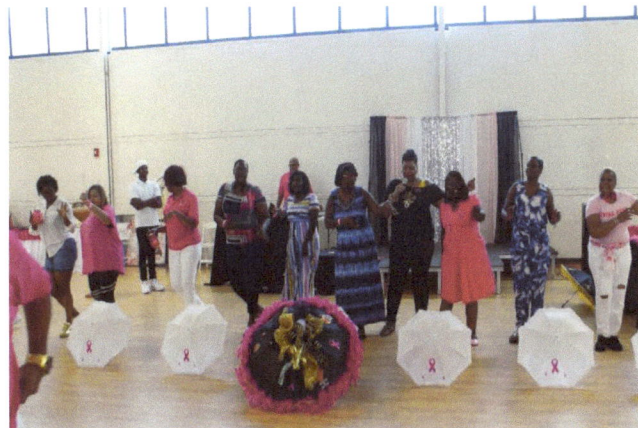

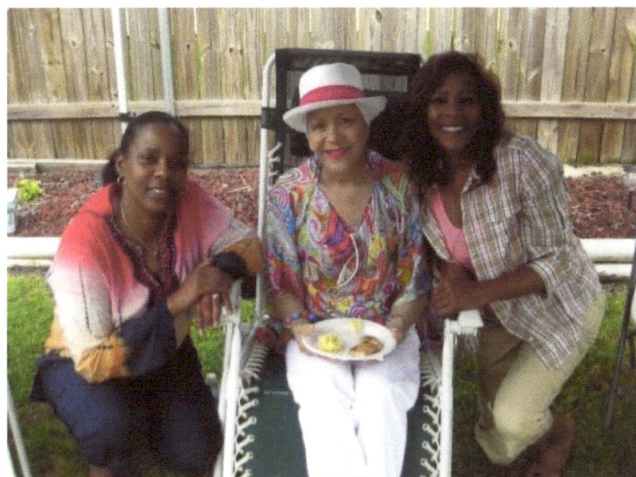

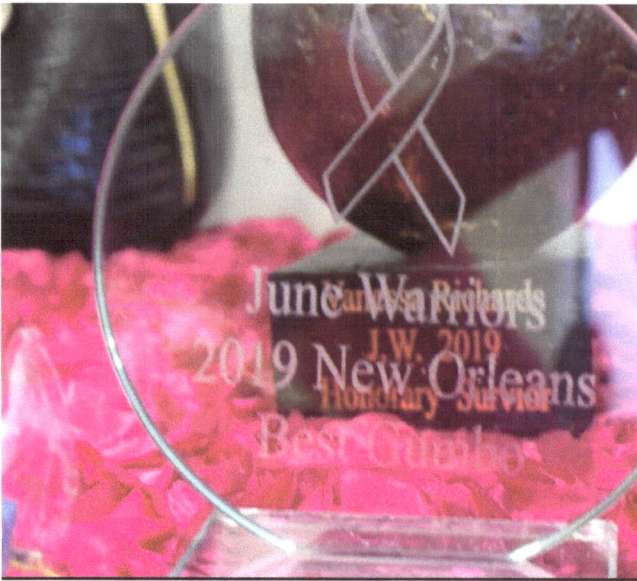

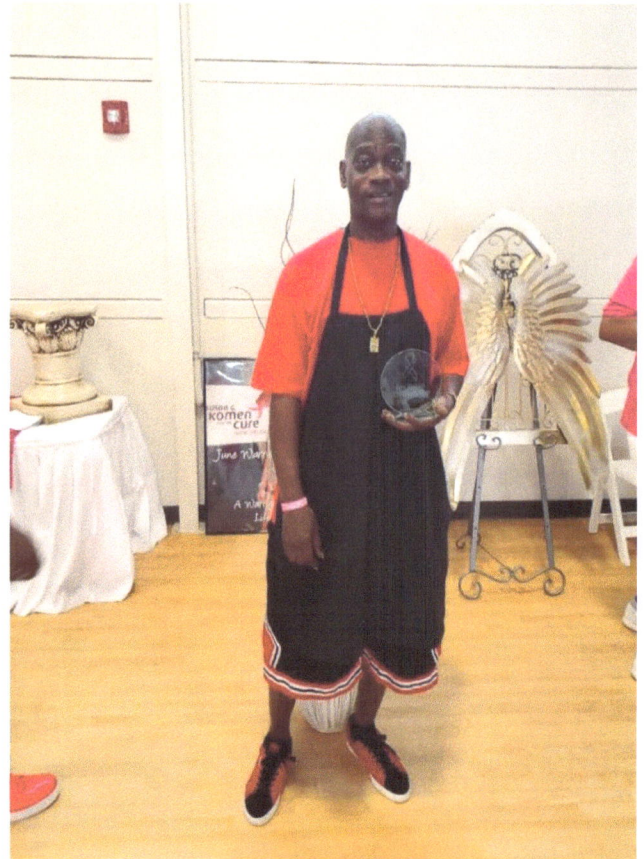

On top: *Award for the Gumbo competition at the survivor event 2019. John Lewis took first place for best New Orleans Gumbo 2019.* Below: *The future, our young advocates supporting the cause. Advocating hope.*

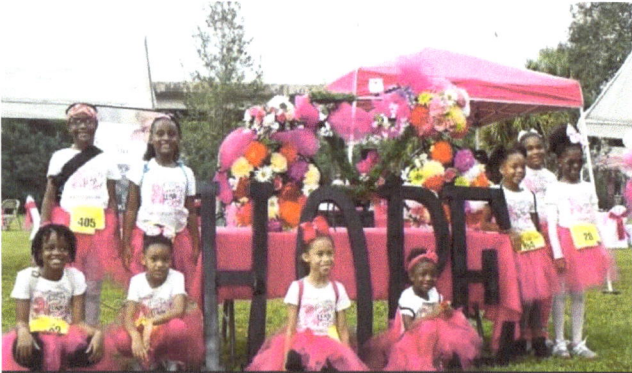

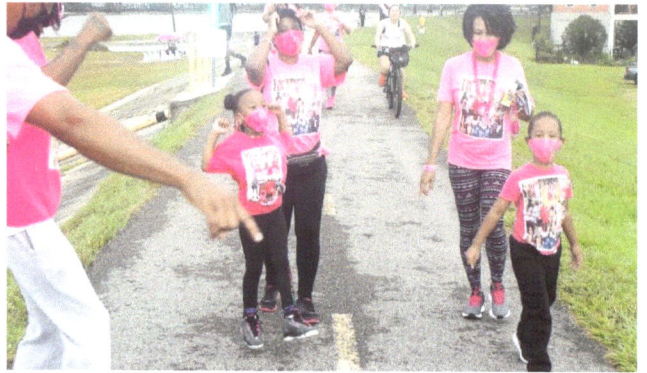

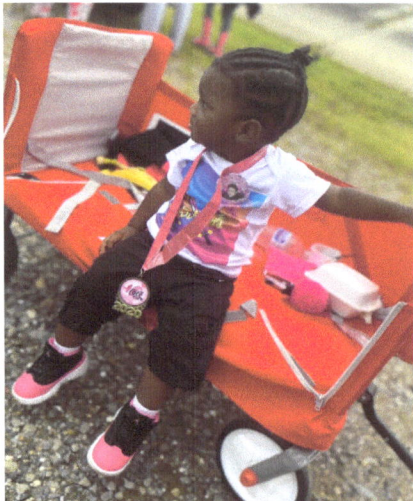

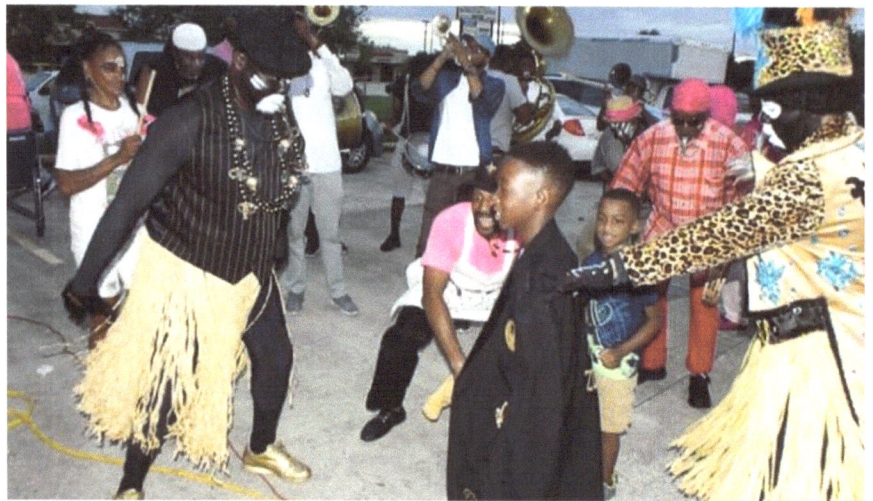

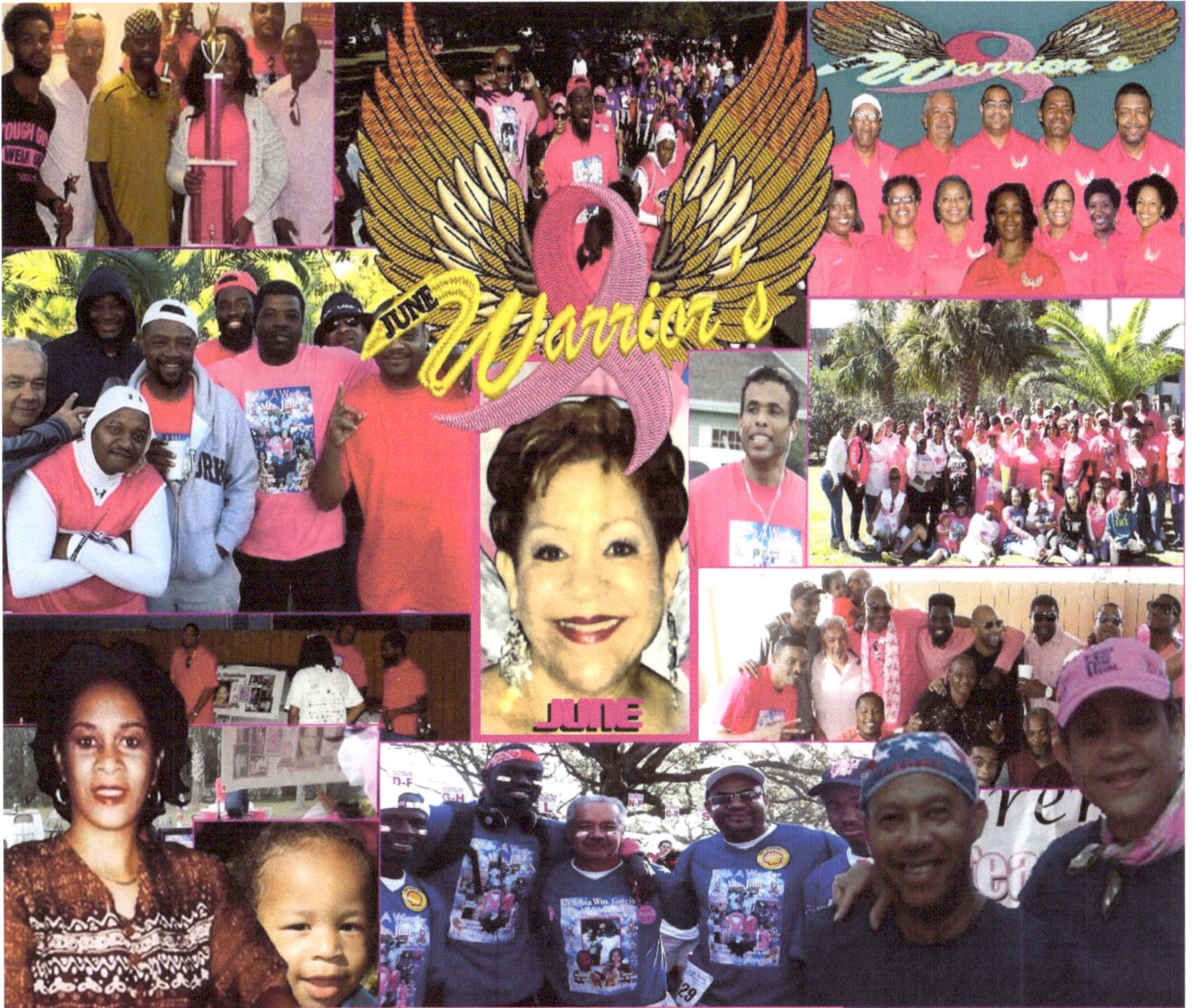

LIFE OF A WARRIOR
Keeping The Promise

Our Warriors believe you live by Hope, because without Hope and Faith you have no focus, no purpose, and giving up is not an option.

NEVER
Give Up
HOPE

A C K N O W L E D G M E N T

God of Victory, I thank you because I know I can do all things through you. It is you who strengthens and guide me. To you, I give all the praise and glory.

Thanks to the June Warriors family for their continuing support and keeping the promise.

Thanks to all of June Warriors supporters, because without you, this would not be possible.

Thank you to The Susan G. Komen New Orleans organization and Lisa Plunkett for the support given throughout the years.

Thanks to Maria Aduke Alabi from Quisqueyana Press publishing company for standing behind our vision and helping with the progress of bringing this book to life.

Thank you to all our Warriors... team members... family and friends.

Together We Can!!!

Given up is not an option, and one day there will be a cure. We won't stop fighting until we find a cure for cancer. Continue to tell your stories.

Let your light shine!!!

Demetris Price

AFTERWORD

We hope this book encourages and inspires those who are fighting this awful disease. Never give up hope, you are not alone. There are all kinds of resources, Susan G. Komen, St. Jude Children's Research Hospital, Kingsley House, The Gayle and Benson Cancer Center, and MD Anderson Cancer Center.

Know your risk. Early detection saves lives.

The Top 5 deadliest cancers

- Prostate cancer.
- Pancreatic cancer.
- Breast cancer.
- Colorectal cancer.
- Lung cancer.

A majority (61.6%) of respondents perceived cancer as death sentence, and more than one-third (36%) of respondents reported they avoid seeing their physicians. In the adult US population, perceiving cancer as a death sentence is wrong. It's not a death sentence and we are here to give you testimony and see God's miracles. Our survivors are winning this battle and kicking cancer's butt. Help us find a cure for cancer, tell your story, give that hope to someone who may be struggling with this.

June Warriors

ADVOCATES FOR THE CURE FOR CANCER

Keeping the promise

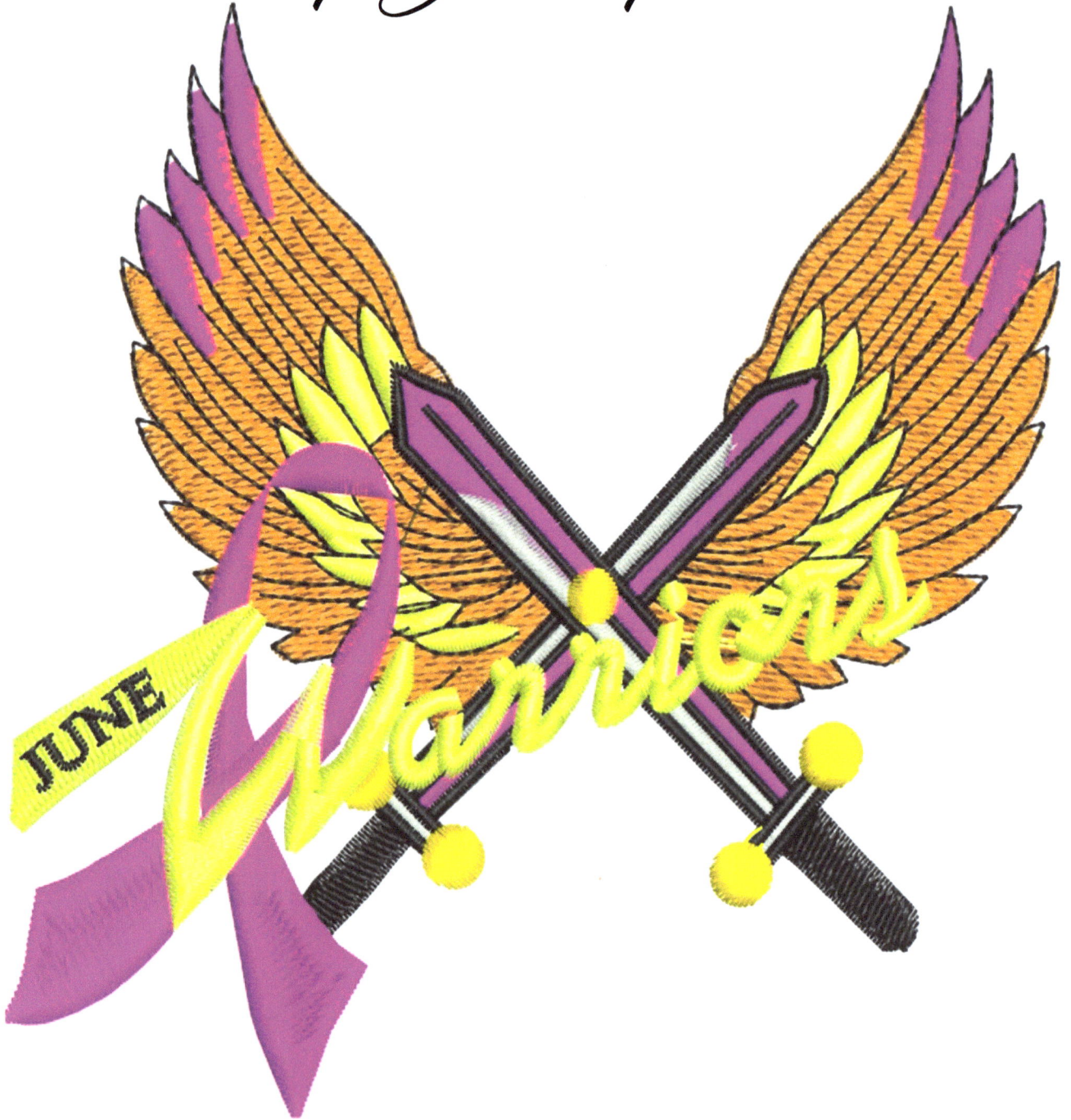

C A L L   T O   A C T I O N

FOLLOW June Warriors on Facebook group **@June Warriors**

For DONATIONS to our non-profit organization, please:

Scan to donate with Cash App

$JuneWarriors

90% of all the proceeds made are always taken in by June Warriors to the organizations for cancer research and Susan G. Komen to organization for research to find a cure for cancer, the other remaining 10% of proceeds go into helping us be able to give the events around the city.

If you enjoy the book
and consider it is a helpful piece to create awareness about cancer not being a death sentence, please help us. Leave your REVIEW on Amazon.

FOR PURCHASE OR MORE INFORMATION ABOUT THIS BOOK AND THE AUTHOR VISIT:

WWW.QUISQUEYANAPRESS.COM/DEMETRIS-PRICE

www.ingramcontent.com/pod-product-compliance
Lightning Source LLC
Chambersburg PA
CBHW061140030426
42335CB00002B/54